HOMEOPATHIC

REPERTORY, CASE TAKING, AND CASE ANALYSIS

METHODOLOGY

An Introductory Homeopathic Workbook

Todd Rowe, MD

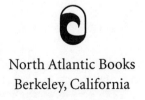

North Atlantic Books
Berkeley, California

Homeopathic Methodology

Published by
North Atlantic Books
P.O. Box 12327
Berkeley, California 94712

Cover and book design by Legacy Media, Inc.
Printed in the United States of America

Homeopathic Methodology is sponsored by the Society for the Study of Native Arts and Sciences, a nonprofit educational corporation whose goals are to develop an educational and crosscultural perspective linking various scientific, social, and artistic fields; to nurture a holistic view of arts, sciences, humanities, and healing; and to publish and distribute literature on the relationship of mind, body, and nature.

Library of Congress Cataloging-in-Publication Data
Rowe, Todd, 1958–
    Homeopathic methodology : repertory, case taking, and case analysis : an intoductory homeopathic workbook / Todd Rowe.
        p.   cm.
    ISBN 1-55643-277-1 (alk. paper)
    1. Homeopathy—Case studies.   2. Homeopathy—Problems, exercises, etc.   I. Title.
    [DNLM: 1. Homeopathy—methods.   WB 930 R879h 1998]
RX75.R69 1998
615.5'32—dc21
DNLM/DLC
for Library of Congress   98-17727
                                                                                      CIP

2 3 4 5 6 7 8 9 10 / 02 01

An Introductory Homeopathic Workbook

Foreword

The needs of beginning homeopaths have long been ignored. A new practitioner is simply supposed to catch on to the whole science or to begin a lengthy course on homeopathy before knowing what it's all about. The present work by Todd Rowe changes all that.

Dr. Rowe has created the finest introductory text to date. It covers the practical aspects of case taking and analysis thoroughly and with insight. The intimidating tools used by homeopaths—repertories and materia medicas—are made accessible by Dr. Rowe's careful step-by-step guidance.

This fine contribution to our literature will make the training of new homeopaths more rapid and less painful. It is modern in terminology, making our older homeopathic texts more comprehensible. Furthermore, Dr. Rowe has given a rounded and clear general introduction to new trends in homeopathy, integrating the insights of Vithoulkas and Sankaran into an overview of classical homeopathy. The book fulfills a glaring void in our literature.

Roger Morrison M.D.
Berkeley, California
January 1998

Acknowledgments

I would like to thank the following people for their tremendous contributions in editing this workbook:

Lesley Hesselmann, Jean Hoagland, Thelma Rowe, Psy.D., Betty Wood, M.D., and Michael Schaeffer.

I also obtained invaluable assistance from Bill Mann, L.Ac., Paul Mittman, N.D., Eilleen Nauman, D.H.M. (UK), Ilene Spector, D.O., Sara Cota, and Dana Ullman, M.P.H.

I am deeply grateful to all of my teachers without which this work would be impossible: Bill Gray, M.D., Nancy Herrick, P.A., Vicky Menear, M.D., Roger Morrison, M.D., Rajan Sankaran, Jonathan Shore, M.D., and George Vithoulkas.

My thanks go to David Warkentin, P.A. for the usage of the McRepertory program through out the workbook. *The Dictionary of Homeopathic Terminology,* by Jay Yasgur, R.Ph., was of great assistance. Ann Seipt, N.D. provided invaluable help with the appendices. Lastly, the new translation of the *Organon,* edited by Wenda Brewster O'Reilly, Ph.D., was used throughout this work and is a wonderful addition to the homeopathic literature.

I would also like to express my appreciation to the many others who contributed their time and effort to this project.

Introduction

There are said to be three pillars of studying homeopathy. These are repertory, case taking, and materia medica. This workbook will address the first two facets.

This is an introductory level homeopathic workbook. Usage of this workbook presupposes an understanding of the fundamentals and principles of homeopathy. There are concepts that are used in this workbook that can only be fully understood by this knowledge. *The Science of Homeopathy* (see below) provides a good overview of homeopathy.

The goals of this workbook are twofold. The first is to create a resource tool for study groups and for homeopathic educators teaching introductory homeopathy. The second is to help individuals take the next step in their own homeopathic education.

There are a variety of appendices to this book. These were written to make working through the body of the text easier. You may want to familiarize yourself with these prior to beginning the text. A glossary of terms is included in Appendix M.

Throughout the book, the *Organon* of Samuel Hahnemann is cited. The translation comes from the 6th edition, edited by Wenda Brewster O'Reilly.

Required Textbooks:
1. *Repertory of the Homeopathic Materia Medica* by James Tyler Kent
2. *Pocket Manual of Homoeopathic Materia Medica* by William Boericke

For More Information:
1. *Complete Repertory* by Roger Van Zandvoort
2. *Concordant Materia Medica* by Frans Vermeulen
3. *Desktop Guide to Keynotes and Confirmatory Symptoms* by Roger Morrison, M.D.
4. *A Dictionary of Homeopathic Terminology* by Jay Yasgur
5. *Science of Homeopathy* by George Vithoulkas
6. *Spirit of Homeopathy and Substance of Homeopathy* by Rajan Sankaran
7. *Synthetic Repertory* by H. Barthel, M.D. and W. Klunker, M.D.
8. *Organon of the Medical Art* edited by Wenda Brewster O'Reilly, Ph.D.

Table of Contents

LESSONS

Casetaking Practical Aspects, PART ONE

Introduction

It has been said that a case well taken is a case half-cured. Casetaking is one of the central pillars on which homeopathic practice stands. A good case stands out and calls out the remedy. Consistent and reliable prescribing comes from the ability to take a good case. Lack of success in homeopathic prescribing is most often associated with poor casetaking rather than a lack of knowledge of materia medica or an inability to properly analyze the case.

There is no right or wrong way to take a case. Casetaking is unique to the individual. It is something that continuously evolves, even after many years of practice. There is always a next step to better casetaking. The best way to learn casetaking is to practice it. Observation of professional homeopaths taking cases is also helpful.

In the *Organon* Aphorism 83 Hahnemann describes the keys to casetaking: "This individualizing examination of a disease case…demands nothing of the medical arts practitioner except freedom from bias and healthy senses, attention while observing and fidelity in recording the image of the disease."

First Aid/Acute/Constitutional

First aid is emergency aid or treatment given to someone injured or suddenly ill, often before medical services can be obtained. Generally, the condition comes on suddenly and violently.

The allopathic definition of acute is a crisis of severe symptoms, having a short course with a prodrome (forewarning) and a zenith, which is self-limited by cure or death. The homeopathic definition of acute is a self-limited illness with symptoms of a different character from the patient's usual illness. These symptoms are stronger and have more distinguishable characteristics or modalities. During the acute crisis the chronic symptoms usually go into remission. Acute diseases arise from specific causes cooperating with susceptibility. When there is an epidemic, only some people get sick, even though most people are exposed to the bacteria or virus. This is caused by the innate resistance or lack of susceptibility in certain people.

The allopathic definition of chronic is a series of symptoms that persist for a long time with very little or extremely slow progression. The homeopathic definition of chronic is a period of prodrome followed by a period of progress that can be quiescent but when aroused leaves the patient worse than before and with no tendency to recover if untreated. Hahnemann felt that most chronic diseases stem from the presence of miasms (see Lesson Ten).

Casetaking is similar for all three types of prescribing. What differentiates first aid casetaking, acute casetaking, and constitutional case taking is the depth and intensity with which the case is pursued. The difference is in degree and not in kind. First aid cases can generally be taken within a matter of minutes. An acute case often takes 15–25 minutes to complete. A constitutional case will take from 90–120 minutes.

In acute casetaking, the intention is to find the totality of symptoms that are departures from the constitutional state. The goal is to accelerate the process of healing and to reduce the risk of any lingering effects from the illness. Acute casetaking is often somewhat easier than constitutional casetaking because the symptoms are fresher and more vivid in the patient's mind. Hahnemann states in Aphorism 82: "Some distinction is to be made between sufferings that are acute, rapidly arising diseases and those that are chronic. In acute diseases, the principal symptoms become more rapidly conspicuous and discernible to the senses so that a much shorter time is needed to note down the disease image. Since most of the acute disease presents itself spontaneously, there is much less that needs to be asked. Gradually advanced chronic disease of several years duration are discovered far more laboriously."

Occasionally, acute cases can be confused with constitutional cases. For example, consider a case of a young man with chronic migraine headaches. A particular episode of the headaches are treated acutely with a resolution of symptoms, but then the headaches recur. A better treatment would be to take the constitutional case, treating the whole person and curing the underlying condition. With a case that is a mixture of acute and constitutional symptoms or is unclear, it is best to treat the person constitutionally or to wait until the case becomes more clear. The best prescription is often to wait.

Observation

One of the most critical aspects of good casetaking is careful observation. This has been much neglected in allopathic medicine. Medical doctors are taught to rely far more on laboratory studies or sophisticated diagnostic imaging techniques than the powers of careful observation. This was the one skill, coupled with the "power of deduction," that brought Sherlock Holmes to the level of greatness. In cases of children or cases of adults who cannot talk, careful observation may be the only way of uncovering the case.

Observation is defined as the act of perceiving or noticing. It involves not only paying attention to what is presented, but also to how it is presented. It is not just the song, but also the dance. We need to listen to the language that the patient uses.

What are the words that stand out or come up over and over in the case? What is their tone of voice? How do they communicate with you? How open or closed are they with you? How do they react to your presence? What is the quality of their emotions or mood? Is their affect congruent with their mood (some people may smile, representing their affect in the moment, but you sense that behind that smile is much sadness, representing their underlying mood)? Are they provocative? Are they present with you, or are they dissociated or only partly there? Are they on time?

We also want to observe the physical aspects of the patient. What is the texture or tone of their skin? What is their complexion like? Are their eyes dilated or constricted? Are they neat and well dressed or slovenly? How is their eye contact? What is the quality of their hand shake? How are they breathing? Are they perspiring? If so, where and how much? What kind of movements do they make during the case, and what does this tell you about them? Are they restless? What is their body language saying (some people may say one thing, but their body language is revealing something different on a deeper level)? What is their general energy level like? How is their posture? How do they walk in? What is their gait like? What are they doing when you first greet them? Are they busy doing work or reading *People* magazine? How do they react to the environment? How sensitive are they (e.g., someone who startles at the sound of a distant phone)? Are there any obvious physical abnormalities? What type of clothes are they wearing? What type of colors or patterns are found in their clothes?

It is often the little observations that lead to the prescription of the right remedy. It is important to pay attention to the details. The philosopher Spinoza once said: "God is in the details." Hahnemann states in the *Organon* Aphorism 95:

> Chronically ill patients become so accustomed to their long sufferings that they pay little or no attention to the smaller, often very characteristic accompanying befallments which are so decisive in singling out the remedy. They view them as almost a part of their natural state, nearly mistaking them for health, whose true feeling they have fairly well forgotten during the course of their fifteen to twenty year long suffering. It hardly occurs to them to believe that these accompanying symptoms, these remaining smaller of greater deviations from the healthy state, could have a connection with their main malady.

Observations of oneself as a homeopath are also critical in taking a case.

Setting

It is important to pay attention to the setting of casetaking. Observation in the home environment is helpful, although not always practical. This provides a view of someone in their natural setting, which can give information about the person.

Whatever setting is used, it should be comfortable for someone to talk freely. It is only when someone is comfortable and trusting that they begin to open up and share their innermost thoughts and feelings. The setting must permit them to feel unhurried and listened to. If there is a waiting area, it is best to greet people there. What they are doing while they are waiting gives useful information about them.

The area for the interview should be private. It should be quiet, with minimal distractions. There should be no religious pictures present and no discernible odors. The temperature should be comfortable. It is best to sit directly in front of them if possible. Some homeopaths choose to sit behind a desk, for ease of access to books and repertory. This can have the effect of distancing yourself from the patient.

Another important aspect of setting is your own internal comfort. You should feel comfortable as a homeopath, or you won't be able to successfully take the case. This includes making sure that you are well rested and unhurried. Take as much time as you need. This is particularly important as a beginning homeopath.

How To Begin

There is no right or wrong way to begin. This is very individual and you have to develop your own style. We must have a sense of trust that the vital force will express itself in a way that is best for the patient, if we are open to it. It may be necessary to set them at ease and make them comfortable before you start. With acute case-taking you have to be more directed and focused than with constitutional case-taking. Acute cases are less in-depth because psychological, emotional, and mental factors often play less of a role.

It is best to say very little at the start of a case. The most common mistake for beginning homeopaths is talking too much. Once you get them started, there will be time for more directed questioning later in the interview. Leading questions narrow and shut down what would otherwise come up spontaneously. An example of a leading question would be: "Do you have problems with constipation, yes or no?" The best symptoms in a case are the ones that come spontaneously and without specific questioning. Hahnemann states in the *Organon* in Aphorism #84: "The physician keeps silent, allowing them to say all they have to say without interruption, unless they stray off to side issues." Later in Aphorism #87 he says: "The physician should never be guilty of seducing the patient into giving false answers and making false statements with any leading questions of suggestions."

It is important to convey to someone that you are not only interested in what brings them to you but also who they are as a person. Examples of introductory statements include:

• Tell me both about what brings you here and about yourself.

• Tell me everything.

• Tell me your story.

Chief Complaint

The chief complaint is the main issue or problem that brings someone to see you. It is what is most important to the patient, although it is often less useful in finding the remedy. However, it is important to honor the patient's view of what the problem is.

With the chief complaint, it is helpful to know the modalities that accompany it and how long the problem has been going on. Modalities are factors that modify a particular symptom, often making it better or worse. You can ask, "What makes your symptoms better or worse?" The symptom of "Headache" is not very useful. However, the symptom of a "Bursting headache in the occiput that extends to the right shoulder at nine p.m. that occurs every day," is much more useful. This is because of the accompanying modalities.

Modalities include character (e.g., bursting pain), location (e.g., occiput), laterality (e.g., left-sided), time aggravation (e.g., nine p.m.), weather (e.g., damp rainy weather), and miscellaneous factors (e.g., worse after eating dinner). Unexpected modalities often help lead to the remedy. The stronger the modality, the more useful it is as a symptom. In recording cases, the common convention is that the symbol "less" refers to "made worse by" (aggravates) and the symbol "more" refers to "amelioration by" (e.g., head pain "less" noise).

Searching for concomitants, alternates, and prodromal symptoms is also helpful. Concomitants are symptoms that accompany the main symptom (e.g., head pain accompanied by diarrhea). Alternates are symptoms that alternate with the main symptom (e.g., diarrhea alternating with arthritis). Prodromal symptoms are ones that precede the onset of the main symptom (e.g., zigzags in the vision prior to the onset of a migraine headache).

Another useful idea is that of pace. Some remedy states present themselves slowly and others present themselves rapidly. It is usually not necessary to get all the details of the progression of the illness over time. What has occurred with the symptoms in the last few days, however, is often quite useful.

Causation/Etiology

Causation, or etiology, is a critical factor in casetaking. It is important to know what was going on at the time of onset of the problem. This could have been a physical, emotional, or mental stress. Changes in jobs, changes in relationships, significant changes in their life, or grief are common factors. Often patients don't initially remember but when pressed will be able to recall. A useful question is "What was going on at the time that the problem started?" and "How did you feel about it?"

Mental/Emotional Symptoms

Mental and emotional symptoms are often the most important symptoms in a case. Much of this will come up from the free flow of the case as they tell their story or through your observations. For acutes, a useful question is "How has your mental and emotional state changed since the onset of the illness?" The simple statement "Tell me about yourself" is often enough to get much of this started.

In constitutional casetaking, when the above is not enough, there are some useful questions to consider asking. These include:

- What do you love most about life?
- What concerns do others express about you?
- What are you teased most about?
- What bothers you the most about other people?
- What are you the most sensitive to?
- How do you feel about yourself?
- Where do you feel the most limited in your life?
- What don't you tell other people?
- How do you handle stress?
- What have been the most significant events in your life, and how did they affect you?

Finding out what their life was like growing up provides insights into this area. This represents a time before they became more well defended when you can better see their natural state. How they handle themselves when significantly stressed is similar, because their defenses are weakened at that time and the natural state becomes more apparent. In women, the premenstrual state often represents such a time, when their underlying state is aggravated due to hormonal stress.

Often what we are looking for is unusual emotional content associated with the condition. For example, it is not unusual for them to be irritable when ill, but to feel rage at anyone talking to them at that time is characteristic. It is also useful to observe their thought processes. How is their mental clarity, their concentration, and their memory? Do they get distracted easily?

There are several specific areas that are helpful to cover, particularly in constitutional casetaking. The first is that of fears. Fears are often a window into what lies deeper in the unconscious of an individual. The questions "Tell me about your fears" or "What do you worry about?" are useful, but often not enough. Many people forget that they have fears or won't own up to them without prodding (particularly men). It is useful to list a series of common fears such as heights, crowds, narrow places, animals, dark, death, public speaking etc., to see if any of these resonate. The most common fear is that of public speaking (40 percent of people), while the deepest fear is often that of death.

Another important area is that of dreams. Freud called dreams the royal road to the unconscious. Here again, these often must be pursued with some prodding. Often the dream they have the night before they come to see you is critical and represents a gift that their unconscious is bringing to you. It is important to find out not only what the content of the dreams are, but the emotion as well. Recurring dreams are important and often represent unresolved conflicts in the individual's psyche. Recurring themes in the dreams are similar. Asking about dreams that occurred at the onset of symptoms can be helpful in understanding the causation or etiology in a case. Dreams are best asked about at the point in the case where there is the deepest emotional content. Looking at the dreams at this point is a method to go deeper at that time.

The emotional state around the time of the period (menses) is often quite helpful. Often this is an exacerbation of the underlying emotional state. Menopausal emotional and mental changes are also important to explore.

The nature and quality of our relationships say much about who we are. Often our deepest desires and conflicts become manifest in the way which we conduct our relationships. Useful questions include:

- What is the quality of your relationships?
- How would you like to change them?
- When did the love die in your life?

Strange/Rare/Peculiar

What we are looking for in casetaking are strange, rare, and peculiar symptoms. These are symptoms that speak to the individual and are not common symptoms typical for the particular pathology. Acute cases (e.g., a cold) can be difficult for this reason, because it may be hard to find the peculiar symptoms in a case. Sometimes this requires relentless pursuit until you find what is individuating about a particular case.

A related issue is to separate what symptoms are common to the situation of the patient from what is unique and peculiar to the individual. This requires a knowledge of the culture and social backgrounds of our patients. Strange/rare/peculiar symptoms arise prior to the onset of any particular situation or pathology. An example might be a Native American patient who comes into my practice for help and says extremely little. This might be taken as reserve or shyness in our culture but is common to the Native American culture. Rajan Sankaran in *The Spirit of Homeopathy* states: "We have to disregard in the patient's mental makeup those features which are due to his socio-cultural environment. We have to remove from the picture all symptoms which are common to the group he belongs to, and which can be explained by his background. What is left is the pure picture upon which you can base a very sure prescription."

Sexuality

The reproductive system is an important area because it reflects the general health of the organism. Issues to explore with female patients include menstrual symptoms (regularity, amount of flow, pain, onset), premenstrual symptoms, pregnancies, infertility, abortions, infections, and menopausal symptoms.

Sexual symptomatology is perhaps best explored near the end of the interview, when more trust and comfort have been established. Some homeopaths do not delve into this area due to lack of comfort. This is unfortunate because it often provides important clues to the remedy. Patients who are the opposite sex from the homeopath often have the most discomfort in this area. My experience is that patients are often more comfortable in this area than we think. Gentle persistence is often the best approach. When a sexual partner is present for the interview, this may preclude honesty in this area. Useful questions include:

- How is your sexual desire and sexual energy?
- How does the sexual energy of you and your partner differ?
- Is there any sexual discomfort or pain?
- Are their problems with impotence?
- How do you feel about sex?
- Is there any history of venereal disease?
- Are you satisfied with your sex life?

Interpretation of sexual desire is subjective. In the Woody Allen movie *Annie Hall,* there is a scene where Woody Allen is asked by his psychiatrist how often he has sex and he responds, "Oh, I never have sex, only three times per week". Another scene shows his partner Annie with her psychiatrist, who asks the same question. She responds, "We have sex all the time, three times per week."

Sleep

Sleep is another area that reflects the general health of the patient. Dreams are covered above in the emotional/mental section. Useful areas to explore are sleep position, refreshing quality of the sleep, drooling, grinding teeth, restlessness, perspiration, sleeplessness, deep vs. light sleep, talking and walking in sleep, sounds made during sleep, movements, desired temperature during sleep, covers, desire to stick body parts out of the covers (e.g., feet or arms), and the emotional state on waking.

Perspiration

Perspiration is particularly useful in acute situations. Areas to explore include quantity, unusual odor, location, time of day, and suppression (e.g., ailments from suppressed perspiration).

Foods/Thirst

Food desires and aversions are helpful in casetaking. It is important to distinguish between what are the natural cravings and what someone thinks is good for them. The latter are useless as symptoms. One way to get at this is to ask, "What must you always keep on the shelves at home and cannot do without?" or, "What foods are hardest to give up on a diet?" Specific food cravings and aversions that can be helpful to ask about include sweets, salt, sour foods, spicy foods, dairy, meat, stimulants, and eggs.

Food aggravations or food sensitivities are also helpful. Alcohol and tobacco usage are important. Thirst is often an important issue. What do they crave in the way of fluids? What temperature do they like their fluids? How is their thirst?

Notes for Lesson One

Quiz for Lesson One

1. Which of the following is not true of acute casetaking?
   - A. A crisis of severe symptoms
   - B. May have a prodrome
   - C. Short course
   - D. Tendency to slowly progress over time
   - E. Self-limited by cure or death

2. What type of questioning is best to begin a case?

3. List four types of modalities that would be helpful in evaluation of the chief complaint.

4. Which of the following is the most common fear?
   - A. Heights
   - B. Crowds
   - C. Insects
   - D. Public Speaking
   - E. Death

5. Which of the following is a strange/rare/peculiar symptom?
   - A. Vaccinosis
   - B. Headache during the full moon
   - C. Allergy to milk
   - D. Suicidal disposition
   - E. Shaking of the extremities during a seizure

6. List four aspect of an individual's sleep that might be helpful in evaluating the case.

(Answers to the quizzes are found in Appendix K.)

Casetaking Practical Aspects, PART TWO

Generalities

The Generalities section covers symptoms that refer to the whole person rather than to a particular part. A number of specific areas should be explored.

Temperature is important. In acute situations this refers to the patient being chillier or warmer than their usual state. In constitutional casetaking this means being chillier or warmer than other people. Often this changes significantly at the time of menopause. Are there particular areas of their body that get cold or hot? Are they bothered by extremes in temperature? Are there particular weather sensitivities? What weather do they most like and dislike?

Another approach is to have them describe an ideal day. What type of climate do they most like? Do they prefer the desert, the ocean, or the mountains? How do the seasons affect them? How are they affected by wind, humidity, sun, or drafts?

How is their energy? What time of day is this at its lowest and highest? How sensitive are they? What are they the most sensitive to? Are there specific sensitivities to noise, light, motion sickness, or odors? How are they with clothing? Do they like it tight or loose, and where on the body? How do they feel about bathing?

Vaccinations are worth inquiring about. What type of reactions have they had to vaccinations in the past? Vaccinations cause both acute and chronic symptoms, which can be an important etiology in determining the correct remedy.

Review of Systems

Review of Systems refers to taking each organ system and asking specific questions about the area. This is less important in acute casetaking. This can be a very time-consuming process and is usually not that helpful in eventually finding a remedy. However, one useful approach is to give them a form to fill out in advance of the interview as a checklist (see Appendix B for a sample questionnaire). Whatever symptoms are checked on the form could then be explored further during the session.

Specific systems include skin (e.g., eruptions, discoloration, hair, nails), the nervous system (e.g., headaches, tremor, tics, restlessness), the digestive system (e.g., stomach pains, indigestion, constipation/diarrhea, hemorrhoids), the musculoskeletal system (e.g., arthritis, pain, weakness, stiffness, movements), the urinary system (e.g., infections, stones, discoloration, frequency, incontinence), the special senses (e.g., hearing, smell, taste, diminished vision or acute vision), the respiratory system (e.g., asthma, difficulty breathing), the endocrine system (e.g., goiter, hyperthyroidism), and the circulatory system (e.g., palpitations, chest pain, cyanosis).

Past Medical History

Past medical history is helpful. Areas to explore include their health as a child, reactions to immunizations, past hospitalizations, surgeries, trauma (especially head trauma), and significant medical problems in the past. Allergies should be identified. Trauma during childbirth is also useful.

Family History

Family history can be simple or detailed. A checklist can save time during the session (see Appendix C for a sample questionnaire). What is important are themes or patterns in the family history. Often these patterns indicate evidence of an underlying miasm (see Lesson Nine). Important areas to explore are a history of tuberculosis, asthma, allergies, venereal disease, mental illness, or heart disease.

In difficult cases where I am not finding the remedy, I will often interview the family separately. Spouses can offer valuable insights into the character and nature of their spouse. This can be done by letter or phone if they are unable to make it in to see you.

Another aspect of family history that can be helpful is the situation of the parents during pregnancy or conception. The emotional/mental state is often transferred to the fetus, even if the parents do not continue in this state. In certain instances, this information can be very helpful in finding the right remedy.

Medications

Medications are always important to ask about. You need to know what conventional medications, over-the-counter medications, vitamins, herbs, and minerals they are taking. The time schedule of the medication is important, in that often medications run out after a certain time with a resultant return of symptoms. If you do not know this, you might misinterpret that there is a specific time aggravation for the symptoms. It is also useful to know what the side effects of particular medications are, as these are symptoms that should not be prescribed upon. Medications can also mask symptoms that would otherwise be there in their natural state, making it more difficult to take a case. Side effects of common drugs can be found in many books such as the *Physician's Desk Reference,* although this is overly inclusive of every possible side effect. Psychoactive drugs should be inquired about. These drugs can interfere/antidote the homeopathic remedies, cause side effects and mask the underlying symptoms. Hahnemann states in Aphorism 91 of the *Organon:*

> The befallments and condition of a patient during some previous course of medication do not give the pure image of the disease. On the other hand, symptoms and ailments suffered before the use of the medicine or several days after discontinuing its use give the genuine, fundamental concept of the original gestalt of the disease…

It is also helpful to know what type of homeopathic treatment they have had in the past. You need to know what remedies they took, what potencies, and what type of response that they had. Knowing what has worked in the past may have a signficant influence on the future usage of that remedy or related remedies.

Obstacles to Cure

Another important factor in casetaking is evaluating for possible obstacles to a cure. These would include things such as stimulant usage, diet, living habits, exposure to things that they are particularly sensitive to and emotional aggravating factors. Unless these obstacles to treatment are removed, homeopathy can produce only a partial response at best. Hahnemann states in Aphorism 94 of the *Organon:*

> While inquiring into the state of a chronic disease, carefully ponder and scrutinize the particular affairs of the patient to find out what there is in them that may arouse or maintain disease and whose removal may further recovery.

Center of Gravity

When the case is complete, it is useful to evaluate the center of gravity of the case. The center of gravity is defined as the place where the majority of the symptoms seem to lie. This is usually described as being on the *physical* level, *emotional* level, or *mental* level. The center of gravity has implications in evaluating the vital force and also assessing how someone is doing on follow-up. For example, if the center of gravity in a case shifts from the mental to the physical level after you give a homeopathic remedy, this generally is a good sign and evidence of movement toward greater health and freedom.

Strength of Vital Force

Another area to assess at the end of the case is the strength of the vital force. This is a concept that has been important in vitalistic philosophy for many centuries, but was popularized in homeopathy by George Vithoulkas in the last twenty five years. The vital force is that energy which directs all aspects of life in the organism. It is that which connects the individual with the energy of the universe. When the vital force is absent, the individual is dead. Assessing the strength of the vital force has direct implications on the potency of the remedy chosen, as well as on the expected prognosis for the case.

The strength of the vital force can be assessed based on five factors. These include the center of gravity (center of gravity on the physical level implies a higher vital force), age (older individuals generally have a weaker vital force), heredity (a poor genetic inheritance implies a weak vital force), sensitivity (the greater the sensitivities, the weaker the organism), and suppression (the greater the amount of suppression by medication or past treatment, the weaker the vital force).

Recording the Case

There are many ways of recording the case. Some homeopaths choose to write very little, and others record nearly a verbatim transcript. Whatever you choose, it is important to be able to bring back the case in your mind by reviewing your notes long after you have recorded the case. Those whose memories are less than excellent often end up recording more. What needs to be recorded are the most important symptoms of the case and also the exact wording of symptoms that are striking or characteristic. Dreams and any unusual language should also be recorded.

It is important to be able to listen and record at the same time. This needs to be done so smoothly that the recording does not interfere with your attention on the case. It is always best to write the case as you are taking it rather than waiting to write it down afterwards. Consistency in your case recording is helpful, so that you will know where to look for things in the future. A well-recorded case is also easily transferable to another homeopath, should this become necessary.

Vital data should be recorded at the start of the case. This should include name, age, telephone number(s), whom to reach in case of an emergency, and observations. An example of an acute case template is included in Appendix A. A standard technique is to leave space after each symptom is initially recorded; then there is room to go back later and fill in the details. Hahnemann states in Aphorism 85 of the *Organon:*

> The physician begins a fresh line with every new symptom or circumstance mentioned by the patient or relation so the symptoms are all ranged separately, one below the other. The physician can

add to any one that is initially stated all-too-indefinitely, but afterwards more clearly.

The physical observations should be recorded at the end of the case. If you are aware of the results of any lab or diagnostic tests, these should be placed here. Next should come your impression. This should include how you assess the case and the most important symptoms to consider in your analysis. Assessment of the center of gravity and vital force can go here.

Lastly should come the plan. This should include the remedy choice, potency, dosing frequency, when they should return, and any other recommendations you make.

Some homeopaths choose to take the case on a computer, while others do it on paper. What is important is what works best for you. In my own practice, I have found that taking the case on the computer allows me to be far more present during the casetaking because I am able to maintain eye contact throughout the entire session. If you choose to take the case on the computer, make sure that you keep a hard copy in case your computer files become damaged.

Underlining

Underlining is a method of bringing a case alive. It helps provide emphasis when you read through a case, like loudness and softness in music. It is a technique that was developed by George Vithoulkas. Once you have done this enough, it begins to become automatic.

Underlining revolves around three keys: clarity, spontaneity, and intensity. Three underlines refer to a symptom that comes up spontaneously, with great clarity and strength. An example of a three underlined symptom is someone who comes in and says "I get this maddening headache that is incredibly severe every day at 3:30 p.m. in my left temple like an ice pick." Two underlines refer to a symptom that is spontaneous but less clear and intense. One underline refers to a symptom that has to be elicited with questioning and is even less clear and intense. How one underlines is individual. Some homeopaths tend to underline more than others. Other factors that influence underlining are peculiarity and frequency. Another technique, used in the same way, is to place (3), (2), or (1) after a symptom in recording a case.

Special Cases

There are certain special cases that require modification of your casetaking technique. Children do not respond to direct questioning in the same way as adults. Watching them play in your office can be helpful. Notice what toys they choose and their style and manner of play. Asking them to draw pictures is often helpful.

After the age of five, it is important that some time be spent alone with the child during the session, although I usually begin with the entire family. It is also helpful to have time alone with the parents, which lets them say things that they don't want to say in front of the child.

Adolescents are often difficult to interview. Taking a successful case hinges on your obtaining their trust. I try to dismiss the parents quickly and make it clear to the teen that this is their treatment. I usually don't see adolescents unless they are at least partially committed to the treatment. Otherwise, they will find some way to sabotage the treatment.

Older patients can be difficult when there are problems with memory and confusion. In cases like this, it is important to get collateral history from their family.

Closed patients are some of the most difficult cases. Symptoms are only given out in a miserly fashion or not at all. You feel like you never really get to know the person, because they won't let you in. In cases like this, collateral history from the family can be helpful. Other areas to explore are their dreams, hobbies, fears, significant events in their lives, their favorite movies and books, occupation, and life passions. These can provide indirect expression of their inner nature. A trusting relationship will permit them to begin to gradually open up over time. Objective observations also become increasingly important in these cases.

Hysterical patients provide the opposite problem. They provide so many symptoms that it is difficult to separate the forest from the trees. Frequently they have a strong anxiety about health, which may lead them from one doctor to the next. What is important for the homeopath here is to stay focused on the center of the case and to not get sidetracked in the myriad of details. Furthermore, it is important to establish a trusting relationship and encourage them to make a commitment to treatment for a specified period of time, before they run off to the next doctor.

Patients who have had much psychotherapy can be difficult. It becomes very hard to separate their therapist's theories of the patient from his or her natural state. In cases like this, it is often helpful to find out what they were like before they started therapy, and what were the issues that brought them in to therapy.

Notes For Lesson Two

Quiz for Lesson Two

1. List four generality areas that are important to cover during casetaking.

2. Where is the center of gravity of the following case?

   J.T. is a five-year-old male who sees you for an acute ear infection. He is shrieking with the pain (2) and quite irritable (3). He cannot make up his mind, asking for something and then pushing it away when he gets it (2). There is a craving for salty foods (2). There is a green diarrhea associated (1).

      A. Physical level
      B. Emotional level
      C. Mental level

3. List four factors that are helpful in determining the strength of the vital force.

4. List three factors that are helpful in determining underlining of a case.

5. John develops a strong craving for pickles (3) after he starts taking the medication Inderol, prescribed for his high blood pressure by his family doctor. He has never had this craving before. Would the symptom "Desires Pickles" be a useful symptom to consider when taking his case?

6. List five systems that might be considered during a Review of Systems?

7. What is an obstacle to cure?

Casetaking Theoretical Aspects

Introduction

Hahnemann calls the process of casetaking "tracing the picture." In his book *The Spirit of Homeopathy*, Rajan Sankaran refers to the process as more one of "Case Uncovering" or "Case Discovering."

The best way to learn casetaking is to practice. It is also useful to watch other homeopaths, observing their style, pace, and approach. Many homeopathic educators use video cases in their teaching to illustrate aspects of casetaking. Ultimately however, you must develop your own style.

The first interview is the most important. It is something that one refers to repeatedly during the course of treatment and that serves as a guidepost from which treatment springs.

When you begin casetaking, it is better to analyze the case after you have taken it. Your mind must be free from prejudice. If you start thinking about a particular remedy too early during the process of casetaking, you limit the myriad of other possibilities and end up proving to yourself your idea. Each case is completely unique. James Tyler Kent says in *Lectures on Homeopathic Philosophy*:

> Keep that in your mind, underscore it half a dozen times, with red ink, paint it on the wall, put an index finger on it. One of the most important things is to keep out of the mind, in an examination of the case, some other case that has appeared to be similar. If this is not done your mind will be prejudiced in spite of your best endeavors. I have to fight that with every fresh case I come to. I have to labor to keep myself from thinking about things I have cured like that before, because it would prejudice my mind.

Jost Kunzli, a twentieth-century homeopath, wrote:

> There is no place for routine, for laziness, for fixed ideas. What is needed is an open mind, sharp intellectual thinking, a very acute sense of observation and a good memory. As long as Homeopathy is practiced in this way, a golden future is assured to her.

Linear, Circular, and Transcendent Thinking

Homeopathy is both an art and a science. This also applies to casetaking. Hahnemann describes the homeopath as a "practitioner of the medical arts."

There is a mountain near where I live. Every day there is a steady stream of people who take the main trail up the mountain, like a trail of ants. This by far is the most popular way to hike the mountain. There also is a circumferential trail that goes around the base. This is a much less traveled trail. Each of these trails offers different insights into the mountain. The kinds of hikers that choose one trail or the other are quite different. The hikers that take the trail to the top tend to be competitive, goal-oriented, and driven. The hikers that take the circumferential trail tend to be slower, contemplative, and more friendly.

Much of allopathic medicine, and even homeopathy in the past, has involved linear thinking. Linear thinking is a goal-directed deductive type of thinking. This is the type of thinking that lies behind the scientific method. Homeopaths who work with this type of thought are like scientists, detectives, or archaeologists in their work.

Circular thinking lies behind the artistic method. It involves seeing the whole rather than the parts. Homeopaths who work with this type of thought are like artists, musicians, dreamers, and visionaries.

The best homeopaths embrace both types of thinking. It is the ability to go back and forth between both ways of thinking that leads ultimately to transcendent thinking. Transcendent thinking allows one to go beyond the surface and to perceive directly. In the case of the story above, this would mean direct perception of the mountain. Transcendent thinking, in homeopathic terms, is the ability to perceive the heart of a case and the heart of a remedy.

Intention

In casetaking, intention is an important key. Our intention is to focus on information leading to the remedy. We are trying to understand the person sitting in front of us as deeply as we can, within the time constraints that we have. Some have described this as a "falling into the patient." You have to have the capacity to live the experience of the patient. In this process, there is often a deep connectedness that occurs. Homeopathic patients frequently leave the first interview saying that they feel more understood than by any other healer that they have seen in the past.

This is different from the allopathic intention, which is to make a diagnosis during the initial interview. This is also different from psychotherapy, where the intention is a working through of deep-seated emotional and mental conflicts. At first, the homeopathic process may be confusing for patients who are used to the allopathic model. Once the homeopath reaches this deeper level, she then moves on. Eventually, the patient will pick up on your intention and go with you. We must not stop until everything fits.

Eventually, you get to a place of integration. This comes from the transcendent thinking described above. This is a place where everything fits together, where there is insight into the core issues leading to a deeper understanding of the patient. When you get to this level, a healing energy with a life of its own has been born. Occasionally, there will be an experience of grace where both patient and homeopath are healed. Rarely, there are homeopathic cases where the initial casetaking is all that is needed; the interview in itself is like giving a homeopathic remedy, and a spontaneous healing occurs.

The feeling that must be conveyed to the patient during casetaking is interest and concern. It is precisely this which gives the patient the courage to delve deeper into themselves and share the innermost aspects of themselves.

Perception

Perception is another key to casetaking. In *The Little Prince,* by Antoine de Saint Exupery, the fox tells the Little Prince the secret of his life: "It is only with the heart that one can see rightly; what is essential is invisible to the eye." Perception involves seeing rightly from the heart. Our patients are not just listing symptoms; they are telling us a living, vital story. We must look and perceive a living image of the disease state before us and not just seek data. James Tyler Kent said of this: "You must see and feel the internal nature of our patient as the artist sees and feels the picture he is painting. He feels it. Study to feel the economy, the life, the soul."

Listening With the Third Ear

Not only must the homeopath perceive deeply, but she must also listen in a different way. It is a type of listening that is similar to reading between the lines. It is a listening for what is most important in a case and for what lies beneath the surface. One way to approach this is through the use of language. Often the choice of language provides insights into the case. When a patient uses the same linguistic imagery over and over, this says something about them. Recording the precise words can be helpful, because this communicates the precise sound of what they are saying. Also, the first thing that they say when they see you is often the most revealing thing about the person and the case.

Importance of the Field

We must not only pay attention to the patient, but also to what goes on around us during the interview. This is the energetic field formed by the patient, the homeopath, and their respective intentions. I have had cases where an external event occurred during casetaking that reminded me of a particular remedy, and when I refocused on the case, this was the remedy needed. Carl Jung spoke of this in terms of synchronicity. The universe conspires to give all that is needed if we are open to listening and perceiving in the right way.

Self-Observation

Observation of our own response and feelings in a case can be quite helpful. It is important to value what you experience and feel. Often we respond in particular ways to particular remedies and once we are aware of this in ourselves, we can use this as valid information. For example, I tend to respond to Pulsatilla cases with a desire to nurture and protect. I react to Aurum cases with a feeling of heaviness, seriousness, and a need to cure the case at all costs. Each of us responds differently to different remedies.

Sometimes these reactions interfere with our being able to successfully take or manage a case. This is called countertransference. It is the aspects of ourselves that we are most uncomfortable with, that we are unable to see in others. Carl Jung called this the shadow. The better we know ourselves, the more effective we become as homeopaths.

Another important aspect of self-observation is our dreams. Our dreams can provide important information about a case as well as provide access to a deeper level of understanding. Occasionally I have had cases where I have been at an impasse until a dream revealed how to move forward again.

Judgments

It is critical to take a case without judgment. It is the extent to which we are non-judgmental that allows our patients to fully reveal themselves to us. We must learn to cultivate the attitude of humility. It is not the homeopath that does the healing, nor the remedy. It is always the physician within. Judgments take us out of the space of moving into the patient and place us solely in our heads. As long as we are really listening and perceiving deeply in a case, there will be no judgment.

Performance Anxiety

One of the major blocks to good casetaking is performance anxiety. Performance anxiety is about the pressure to do it right and find the correct remedy. This causes us to tense up, become self-conscious, and move away from the heart of a case. We need to learn to relax into the picture. This involves going to the same place that you might go in prayer or meditation. When the pressure is on is when you most want to relax. This is totally opposite from allopathic thinking.

Techniques to Go Deeper

There are many ways of encouraging someone to go deeper as you are taking a case. Often this occurs simply with the statement: "Tell me more." To the extent that we can, it is best to use nondirective questions and avoid leading questions that prevent this deepening process.

A useful technique is to look for areas of discomfort. This is the area of the wound(s) in the case that the patient is protecting because of the pain. Often there are walls of protection around these areas to isolate and hide them. This wall always has weak spots, and this is where the discomfort pokes through. Focusing on these areas is difficult for a beginning homeopath because there is a natural tendency to avoid the areas that are discomforting. However, it is precisely these areas that allow us to go deepest in a case and to the heart of the problem. It takes courage for both the patient and the homeopath to go after this. Subtle clues can point to areas of discomfort. Changes in body posture, dilation of the pupils, repetitive motions of the extremities, change in voice, and expression of emotion can all indicate this. Commenting on the discrepancy between body language and what they are saying can often lead someone deeper.

There are several types of questions that can be used during casetaking. Lateral questions are ones that are designed to gain information. These are questions about the chief complaint, modalities, food cravings, and body temperature, among others. Often these questions are triggered by the homeopath asking "What else?" Deepening questions are designed to move closer to the heart of the case. These may be triggered by the homeopath asking "Tell me more about…" or "Give me an example of…" Both types of questions are necessary in casetaking.

Cognitive dissonance is an experience where you as the homeopath feel that something is not adding up. This often creates a feeling of discomfort or tension in the homeopath. It represents a paradox where there are two opposing pieces of information. Exploration of this leads to a deepening of the case. It is crucial that you feel comfortable staying within this cognitive dissonance. It often resolves when you find the right remedy.

The last technique to mention is that of pacing. Pacing is an Eriksonian hypnotic technique that involves putting yourself in the same space as the patient physically, generally, and emotionally. This may involve mirroring their body movements or their emotional state. For example, when someone is talking very quietly about something, you may find that your own voice drops to mirror theirs. It is important not to do this in a forced or mechanical way. Most good health care practitioners do this naturally and without thought. During casetaking, when you feel yourself drifting or moving away from the center of the case, pacing can be a helpful technique to help you go deeper.

Notes for Lesson Three

Introduction to the Repertory

What is a Repertory?

A repertory is a place where information is stored or categorized so that it can be retrieved more easily. It is an index of symptoms, with a listing of all of the remedies known to be associated with each particular symptom. This information can be stored in a book format, on software, compact disc, or through a collection of cards (card repertories). The word "repertory" comes from the Latin word *repertus,* which means "to find."

Purpose of the Repertory

The purpose of the repertory is to help you find the right remedy for a given case. It is a tool. The repertory helps to individualize a case to find the right remedy for the right person. It also assists the practitioner find small and rarely used remedies and to link unusual symptoms with the appropriate remedy. There are some cases where using the repertory is crucial to finding the right remedy and other cases where it is much less useful.

History of Repertories

Initially in homeopathy there were no repertories. Hahnemann had only proven a few remedies, and it was possible to remember the symptoms that were associated with each of the known remedies. As further provings were undertaken and homeopathic knowledge increased, it was no longer possible to remember all the symptoms associated with each particular remedy. Repertories became increasingly necessary.

The first repertory was created by Hahnemann in 1805 and was handwritten. It was difficult to use, reflecting more an alphabetical index to the provings, and Hahnemann was never entirely happy with it. The next repertory to come out was written by Clemens Maria Boenninghausen in 1832. It was called *Repertory of Antipsorics* and focused on the importance of modalities (something that makes a particular condition better or worse). Georg Jahr also wrote a repertory in 1835 called the *Symptomen-Codex;* it also was handwritten. This repertory was only based on proving symptoms. Hempel translated Jahr's repertory into English and added to it, creating a much more substantial repertory in 1848. The first French repertory was written by Lafitte in 1844 (*Symptomatologie homoeopathique, ou tableau synoptique de toute la matiere medicale pure.* Vol. I, Paris). Lippe was one of the first homeopaths to add more mental and emotional symptoms to the repertory. His repertory was expanded by Lee, who abandoned the effort when he went blind. Much of Kent's *Repertory* is based on the work of Lee and Lippe. Card repertories were popular in India. There have been more than 125 repertories created. Many are complete repertories, while others focus on only a specific area, such as Boenninghaussen's repertory, devoted only to fever (*Verushch einer homoopathic-schen Therapie der Wechselfieber.* Munster, 1833). These repertories are of varying quality and usefulness.

Modern Repertories

In more recent years efforts have been made to create repertories that are easier to use, which update the archaic language of many of the older repertories. Two of the most important of these are the *Complete Repertory* by Roger Van Zandvoort and the *Synthetic Repertory* by H. Barthel and W. Klunker. Both of these repertories are more expensive, but extensively researched, painstakingly constructed, and well designed. Robin Murphy's *The Homeopathic Medical Repertory* is also popular, although considerably shorter. Many of the newer repertories combine older repertories and add symptoms gained from more recent provings. Electronic versions of repertories are becoming increasingly common. Still, Kent's *Repertory of the Homeopathic Materia Medica* remains the most common repertory used in the world today. This workbook uses Kent's *Repertory* as its main reference.

How is Information Added to the Repertories?

The repertories are incomplete. There is always more information that needs to be added. The repertories are primarily based on symptoms obtained from provings. Another method in which remedies and symptoms are added to the repertory is through cured cases. When homeopaths consistently see a symptom cured by a particular remedy, this may be added to the repertory. You may also see information in the repertory that is based on accidental poisonings. For example, one of the ways that we know about the remedy *Heloderma suspectum* (venom from the lizard Gila Monster) is from bites of the animal on humans and the associated symptoms that develop after the bite. These symptoms are then recorded into the repertory. One of the advantages of electronic homeopathic repertories is that this information can be updated much more quickly and regularly.

Grading of Symptoms

When a proving is completed, the symptoms of that particular remedy are added to the repertory on a graded basis. Symptoms that are very strong, clear, and common are added as threes (3) (usually designated by dark and bold type); symptoms less common and only moderately clear and strong are added as twos (2) (usually designated by italics or plain type with underlining); symptoms that are infrequent and weaker in intensity are added as ones (1) (usually designated by plain type).

For example, on p. 37 of Kent's *Repertory,* you will find the heading of "Disgust." Puls *(Pulsatilla)* and Sulph *(Sulphur)* are listed in bold type for this particular symptom (3). Merc *(Mercurius vivus)* is the only remedy listed in italics (2) and Ars *(Arsenicum album)*, Cimx *(Cimex)*, Coloc *(Colocynthis)*, Mez *(Mezereum)* and Phos *(Phosphorous)* are listed in plain type (1).

Kent's Repertory

Kent's *Repertory of the Homeopathic Materia Medica* was written in 1877. He was more of an organizer of other repertories, and much of his work was based on Lippe's work. However, he also added a great deal of information gleaned from his own experience. Kent's *Repertory* contains 648 remedies. His repertory is perhaps best known for its Mind section, which was more complete than any previous repertory in this area.

General Layout of Kent's Repertory

A particular symptom in a repertory is called a rubric. For example, on p. 63 of Kent's *Repertory* you will find the rubric "Loquacity." On p. 766 you will find the rubric "Difficult Respiration."

Remedies are listed alphabetically for each rubric. Abbreviations are used for each remedy (see Appendix D for a listing of abbreviations associated with each particular remedy). This helps to reduce the size of the repertory.

The general plan of the book is to work from generals to specifics and from the top downwards. The book is based on anatomical divisions (see Appendix E for a listing of each separate section). There are thirty-one separate sections. Take a few minutes to familiarize yourself with the sections of the *Repertory*. Note that there are no sections for systems such as the circulatory system or the nervous system. Symptoms that relate to these systems are sometimes found in the Generalities section. The general format is to work from the top of the body to the bottom. For example, the Head section is followed by the Eye section, the Ear section, and then the Nose section.

One of the largest sections of the *Repertory* is the Mind section, which is at the beginning of the book. The Generalities section lies at the end of the *Repertory*. These two sections are the most important and are used the most in prescribing.

Take a moment to review the Word-Index section at the back of the *Repertory*.

This is quite helpful when you are looking for a particular word that you cannot seem to find.

Structure of Kent's Repertory

Each section of the *Repertory* is alphabetical and each main heading is followed by modifiers (see Appendix F for how these modifiers are structured). This format is the general rubric, followed by side modifiers, time modifiers, modalities, extensions, locations and ending with descriptors. This basic structure is followed over and over again in the *Repertory* and it is important to familiarize yourself with this.

The most difficult section to follow in the *Repertory* is the Head Pain section. If you can follow through this and understand how it is structured, then everything else in the repertory will be easier. The "Head Pain" rubric starts on p. 132 in the Head section which starts on p. 107. You will note that over 500 remedies are listed under the rubric "Head Pain." This is the largest rubric in the *Repertory*. Because this rubric is so large, it is not usually very helpful in finding the right remedy for someone with headaches.

Everything following the rubric "Head Pain" from p. 132 until p. 221 is classified as a subrubric. Subrubrics are *modifiers* or descriptions of the initial rubric (in this case "Head Pain"). The first subrubric after the general rubric of "Head Pain" is "daytime" on p. 132. This is the first of the time modalities. This means a headache that occurs during the daytime. Following this is the subrubric "morning" which again means a headache in the morning.

The next subrubric "in bed," is indented and therefore is a sub-subrubric that modifies the preceding subrubric. This means head pain in the morning in bed. Similarly, all of the following subrubrics until "10 p.m." on p. 133 are modifiers of the subrubric "head pain in the morning." For example the subrubric on p. 133 of "increases and decreases with the sun" means head pain that is worse in the morning and increases as the sun rises and decreases as the sun sets. The time modality section then continues with "forenoon" on p. 133 and finally ends with the subrubric "5 a.m." on p. 135.

The next section of modifiers after time aggravations is *Modalities*. Modalities are basically modifiers or qualities that affect the basic symptom. This section begins on p. 135 with "acids from." This means head pain from eating acid food. The section ends finally on p. 152 with "when yawning."

The next section is *Extensions*. This means a symptom that extends from one place in the body to another. For example, the first extension is "extending to the back" which means head pain extending to the back. The section ends with "zygoma" (cheekbone) on p. 153.

The next section is *Locations*. The first location is "Bones." This means head pain that seems to localize in the bones of the head. This section continues until p. 173 when it ends with "Vertex and Forehead." Note that each location, such as forehead on p. 153, goes through the same cycle of structure as the larger sections including a general rubric (153), followed by side modifiers (154), time modifiers (154–5), modalities pp. (155–158) extensions (158–159), and ending with locations (159–161).

The last section of the "Head Pain" rubric is *Descriptors*. Descriptors are qualities of the pain (see Appendix G). This starts on p. 173 with the subrubric "boring" and ends on p. 221 with "wedge like." Note that for each type of pain the same cycle of general rubric, sidedness, modalities, extensions, and locations continues.

Amelioration and Aggravation

You can assume that everything in the *Repertory* means "worse from" unless "amel" is notated. "Amel" stands for ameliorates and means to make the condition better. Therefore the subrubric "daytime" on p. 132 means a headache worse during the daytime. The subrubric on p. 133 of "amel" means head pain that is less in the morning.

Common vs. Uncommon

As you look through the *Repertory* , you will find that some remedies are much more common than others (see Appendix D). Some remedies were very well proven at the time that the *Repertory* was written, and there is a wealth of information available about them (these are also known as polychrests). Others only came into usage later in the development of homeopathy and are poorly represented in the *Repertory*. Many of the remedies that have been proven more recently such as Saguaro *(Carnegiea gigantea)*, Neon, or Dolphin's Milk *(Lac delphinum)*, are not contained in the *Repertory* at all. Information on newer remedies can be found in proving transcripts or in more recent materia medicas (e.g., *The Synoptic Materia Media Two*, by Vermeulen). Periodically, the more modern repertories are updated with information from the most recent provings.

The most common remedy in the *Repertory* is *Sulphur*. See Appendix D for a listing of the most common remedies found in the *Repertory*.

What is Contained in the Repertory?

The *Repertory* generally represents states of pathology or disease. The most important symptoms used in prescribing a homeopathic remedy are symptoms that are based on disease states. The healthy areas of the individual's life are usually not as helpful in finding the correct remedy. Disease represents limitations of freedom in the individual's life. The following are rubrics listed in the Mind section of the *Repertory*:

Benevolence (9)
Cheerful (10)
Laughing (61)
Tranquility (29)

These represent qualities that become symptoms when they are out of balance in the person's life (limitations of freedom). For example, the rubric "Benevolence" could be used for someone who constantly gives their possessions and money away at the cost of being poor and in continuous ill health.

Confusing Rubrics

Rubrics are sorted using the first word of the rubric, while the remainder of the rubric is used as a modifier. For example, on p. 63 you will find the rubric "Love, Ailments from Disappointed" which actually means ailments from disappointed love. On p. 12, you find the rubric "Clinging, children, of, awake terrified, know no one, scream, cling to those near." This refers to a child who awakens terrified and clings to anyone who is near. The sort is on the word "Clinging."

How Is the Repertory Used?

Cases are seldom solved by using a single rubric or symptom. The process of choosing rubrics and combining these to choose the right remedy is called *repertorization*. Generally between three and ten separate rubrics are chosen to solve a case. Appendix I contains a sample blank repertorization sheet. You may want to make copies of this sheet to use in repertorization. Each rubric chosen is written on the top of the repertorization sheet. The remedies are entered into the corresponding columns as either grade one (1), two (2), or three (3). Finally the numbers are totaled up to see which remedy(s) are best represented in the repertorization. The last step in analyzing a case is to study the materia medica of the most well-represented remedies in the repertorization and to choose one that best fits the case.

Ideal-sized rubrics to choose are often ones that are neither too large or too small. Using rubrics that are too large takes a great deal of time to repertorize and often results in a repertorization that leads only to the most common remedies (polychrests). An example of a rubric that is too large to be useful is the rubric "Head Pain" on p. 132, which contains over 500 different remedies.

Using rubrics that are too small can also create problems. This may result in excluding the right remedy from the field. When a rubric contains ten to twenty remedies, this is generally thought to be ideal-sized. Repertorization can be a time-consuming process. In recent years, the use of computers has made this whole process automated and almost instantaneous.

There is no right or wrong way to repertorize a case. Some homeopaths tend to use many rubrics and others use just a few. Many different strategies may ultimately lead to the selection of the right remedy. Again, what is most important is that the repertory is a tool to suggest to you possibilities for further study of remedies leading to the best remedy selection.

A sample case is as follows: John is a forty three-year-old single male who has had an acute, severe sore throat for the last three days. The pain is markedly worse when swallowing liquids and is only on the left side. The pain is also worse when swallowing warm fluids. There is significant pain in the throat pit. There is a very strong craving for pasta. He says that he is afraid to take any medication for this because it might poison his system. The rubrics that were used in the analysis are as follows:

> Throat, Pain, Swallowing on, Liquid (459)
> Throat, Pain, Left (458)
> Throat, Pain, Swallowing, Warm Drinks (459)
> Throat, Pain, Throat Pit (473)
> Stomach, Desires, Farinaceous (485)
> Fear, Poisoned of Being (46)

You can see the repertorization in Appendix I. The remedy that comes through most strongly is *Lachesis*. *Lachesis* is a remedy that is noted to have severe sore throats that are worse on the left side. One of the keynotes for this remedy is pain that is worse when swallowing liquids. People who need *Lachesis* also tend to be warm and are worse from heat. A single dosage of *Lachesis* 30C was administered, and the symptoms resolved completely in six hours.

How to Choose the Most Important Symptoms

The best rubrics to use are those that most characterize the symptoms of the case. Avoid symptoms that are common for the particular pathology of a case and choose rubrics that are uniquely characteristic of the individual person. Common symptoms of a particular disease do not tell you about the person who has the disease. Homeopaths prescribe for the person and not for the disease. Also, mental symptoms and general symptoms are often more helpful in finding a remedy than physical symptoms are. Common symptoms of various diseases can be found in many medical books, such as *Current Medical Diagnosis and Treatment A Lange Medical Book* by Tierney, McPhee, Papakakis, and Schroeder. Some homeopathic software also has this feature.

For example, when someone has a urinary tract infection, the symptom "pain in the bladder" is common and much less useful than the symptom "pain that is only better when the individual is taking a warm bath." Another example is someone with a migraine headache associated with vomiting. The symptom "head pain with vomiting" is very common in migraines and would be less useful than the symptom "head pain associated with violent twitching of the right eye" (a symptom that is not commonly associated with migraines). Finally, the symptom of "anxiety" is common, whereas the symptom of "fear on waking of something under the bed" is far more characteristic.

Additions

When new information is found about a remedy or new provings are performed, this information is then added to the repertory. This is the reason that many of the more modern repertories are larger than the older repertories. There also are published additions that can be written into the repertory. One example is the *Additions of George Vithoulkas*. Also, remedies can be added to rubrics when we see a particular symptom repeatedly cured in our cases, even if this is not listed in the materia medicas.

How Can I Learn to Use the Repertory More Effectively?

The best way to learn to use the repertory is to practice. The more you look up rubrics and find your way around the repertory, the easier it becomes. Repertorization exercises such as those recommended in the next several lessons can be helpful. Ultimately, however, the best way to learn the repertory is through study of cases. There are also several courses available in the further study of repertory.

Notes for Lesson Four

Quiz for Lesson Four

1. Repertorize the following case and find the best remedy.

   A three-year-old child has had colic pains for the last three months. This occurs every night, waking the child around 3 a.m. However, the child's waking at 3 a.m. had preceded the onset of the colic by three months (Sleep, Waking, Midnight after, 3 a.m. p. 1255). The child is quite irritable and cannot wait to be breast-fed (Mind, Impatience, p. 53). The child is quite sensitive to light, which seems to worsen the irritability and pain (Mind, Sensitive, Light, p. 78). There is a strong craving for spicy foods (Stomach, Desires, Highly seasoned food, p. 485). The stomach pain seems to be much better from warm drinks (Stomach, Pain, Warm Drinks Amel, p. 515).

2. Repertorize the following case and find the best remedy.

   Susan is a twelve-year-old girl who was exposed yesterday to poison ivy while she was outside playing with her friends. The eruptions are yellow and look like hives (Skin, Eruptions, Vesicular, Yellow, p. 1323). The eruptions are only on the face (Face, Eruptions, Vesicles, p. 372). The skin eruptions come on strongly for a while and then disappear when she has diarrhea and then the skin eruptions come back (Rectum, Diarrhea, Alternating with skin eruptions, p. 611).

3. Repertorize the following case and find the best remedy.

   Jane is a thirty-two-year-old female who is three months pregnant. Over the last month she has been experiencing increasing nausea and vomiting (Nausea of pregnancy, p. 509). The nausea is much worse when she moves or drives her car (Nausea, motion, p. 508). The smell of food strongly triggers the nausea (Nausea, food, smell of, p. 507). She is quite anxious about her two-year-old son and husband. Because of her symptoms, she is worried that no one will take care of her family (Anxiety for others, p. 7). She keeps going over in her mind a spontaneous miscarriage that she had during her last pregnancy (Dwells on past disagreeable occurrences, p. 39).

4. Repertories are mostly based on which of the following?
   - A. Pathological symptoms
   - B. Poisoning symptoms
   - C. Proving symptoms
   - D. Cured symptoms

5. Which of the following is the correct order for the structure of Kent's *Repertory?*

    A. Modalities; Sidedness; Time aggravation; Extensions; Locations; Descriptors

    B. Sidedness; Time aggravations; Modalities; Extensions; Locations; Descriptors

    C. Time Aggravations; Modalities; Sidedness; Extensions; Locations; Descriptors

    D. Sidedness; Modalities; Time Aggravations; Extensions; Locations; Descriptors

    E. Time Aggravations; Sidedness; Modalities; Extensions; Locations; Descriptors

6. Which of the following is the correct ordering of the sections of Kent's *Repertory?*

    A. Mind; Face; Head; Abdomen; Generalities

    B. Mind; Generalities; Head; Face; Abdomen

    C. Generalities; Face; Head; Abdomen; Mind

    D. Mind; Head; Face; Abdomen; Generalities

    E. Head; Mind; Face; Abdomen; Generalities

Mind Section of Kent's Repertory

General Layout

The Mind section is one of the largest and perhaps is the most important section of the *Repertory*. Hahnemann states in the *Organon* Aphorism #211:

> In all cases of disease to be cured, the patient's emotional state should be noted as one of the most preeminent symptoms… If one wants to record the true image of the disease in order to be able to successfully cure it homeopathically. The preeminent importance of the emotional state holds good to such an extent that the patient's emotional state often tips the scales in the selection of the homeopathic remedy.

The Mind section contains all of the mental and emotional symptoms. Take a few minutes to leaf through the Mind section on pp. 1–95 and familiarize yourself with the layout.

In the past, homeopathic cases were frequently solved by focusing on physical symptoms. As suppression has increased in relation to allopathic drugging, immunizations, and other suppressive therapies, symptoms have been suppressed deeper and deeper into the organism. This has resulted in the increasing importance of mental and emotional symptoms in helping to find the right remedy.

Cross-Referencing

Cross-referencing is a useful way of making it easier to get around the *Repertory*. For example, alcoholism is listed under the rubric "Dipsomania." If you have trouble remembering this, you can write in your repertory the rubric "Alcoholism, See Dipsomania, p. 36" on p. 1. Other times you may want to write in related rubrics. For example, you can find the concept of "Guilt" under "Anxiety of Conscience" on p. 6 and under "Remorse" on p. 71. If you look at these rubrics, you will find that they contain different remedies. You can cross-reference these rubrics by writing the page number of the other rubric next to each one. This will remind you that there are other remedies to consider for a particular concept than simply the ones in the rubric.

Related Concepts

It is helpful to try to differentiate the subtle differences between related concepts in the Mind section. For example, if you consider the ideas of jealousy and envy, you may at first use these interchangeably. However, if you look at the remedies in the respective rubrics, you will find that they are different. When you are taking a case, when should you use the rubric "jealousy" and when should you use "envy"? Jealousy is usually about a particular person and often has a sexual connotation. A man may be jealous of the way that his wife looks at another man. Envy is more about possessions or things. We may envy another person's car or new computer. Another related concept is greed which can be found under "Avarice."

There are many concepts related to sadness. These include:

Brooding (10)
Despair (35)
Discontented (36)
Discouraged (36)
Grief (50)
Inconsolable (54)
Loathing Life (62)
Morose (68)
Sadness (75)
Sighing (80)
Suicidal Disposition (85)
Weary of Life (92)
Weeping (92)

Sadness is more of an inner state of experience, and can be used as synonymous with depression. Grief relates to a particular loss or separation that occurs from the outside. Grief would be appropriate after the sudden death of a loved one. "Inconsolable" is often related to the concept of Grief. There is also a useful rubric, "Love, Ailments from Disappointed" which really means ailments from disappointed love. There is a gradation of intensity of experience from "Brooding" to "Discouraged" to "Despair" to "Weary of Life" to "Loathing Life" to "Suicidal Ideation." "Brooding" also has the quality of a particular thought pattern associated with the emotion. "Morose" has more of a quality of chronicity and a refusal to see anything positive in life, and is often coupled with irritability. A good example of Morose would be the character Eeyore in the book *Winnie the Pooh* by A. A. Milne. Eeyore is always gloomy, complaining, and never happy.

Concepts related to anger include:

Anger (2)
Censorious (10)

Contradict Disposition to (16)
Contrary (16)
Cursing (17)
Delirium, Raging (19)
Destructiveness (36)
Fight, Wants to (48)
Hatred (51)
Indignation (55)
Irritability (57)
Malicious (63)
Misanthropy (66)
Quarrelsome (70)
Rage (70)
Reproaches Others (71)
Tears Things (87)
Unfriendly Humor (91)
Violent (91)
Wildness (95)

"Irritability" relates more to an inner endogenous experience, whereas "Anger" has more of an external focus. We are usually angry "about" something but "feel" irritable. There is a gradation of intensity of experience from "Unfriendly Humor" to "Irritability" to "Quarrelsome" to "Malicious" to "Hatred" to "Rage" to "Violence." "Misanthropy" is a hatred of mankind. "Indignation" usually has a righteous qual-ity to it and stems from a hurt to one's ego. "Resentment" is more of an anger that is turned inward and is chronically smoldering. "Censorious" refers to being crit-ical of others.

Anxiety is well represented in the *Repertory*. Related concepts include:

Mind, Anguish (3)
Mind, Anxiety (4)
Mind, Cares full of (10)
Mind, Fear (42)
Mind, Frightened Easily (49)
Generalities, Anxiety (1345)
Mind, Monomania (67)
Sleep, Dreams Anxious (1236)
Sleep, Dreams Nightmares (1242)
Mind, Starting (82)
Mind, Superstitious (85)
Mind, Thoughts Tormenting (88)

"Anxiety" is an inner experience of emotion. "Fear" has an external focus. I may feel anxious, but I am fearful of taking an exam. "Anxiety about Health" (7) is an important rubric in the repertory and refers to people who are overly concerned about their health, a common problem in our culture. Related concepts here are "Anxiety, Hypochondriacal" and "Fear of Impending Disease." "Monomania" refers to an exaggerated focus and interest in one particular area or idea to the exclusion of all else. A compulsive person who must wash his hands fifty times daily would fit this rubric. "Anguish" is a deeper state of anxiety that has a component of acute pain and suffering attached to it. With anguish there is also a feeling of helplessness.

Guilt finds its expression in two rubrics in the repertory. These are "Remorse" and "Anxiety of Conscience." "Remorse" is a deeper and more painful state than "Anxiety of Conscience," similar to the difference between "Anguish" and "Anxiety."

There are many rubrics relating to confusion. These include:

Concentration Difficult (13)
Confusion (13)
Dullness (37)
Forgetful (48)
Memory Weakness of (64)
Mistakes (66)
Prostration of the Mind (69)
Senses Dullness of (78)
Stupefaction (84)
Torpor (89)
Unconsciousness (89)

A gradation of intensity of these symptoms might be "Forgetfulness," "Concentration Difficult," "Dullness," "Prostration of the Mind," "Torpor," "Stupefaction," and "Unconsciousness." "Confusion" is usually about having too many thoughts, whereas "Dullness" is about having too few thoughts. The section "Mistakes" refers to people who make mistakes in communicating, i.e., writing, spelling, and speaking, or in perception, i.e., in regard to time or localities.

Workaholism is a common problem in our culture. This can be found in the following rubrics:

Activity Desires (1)
Busy (10)
Hurry (52)
Industriousness (56)
Irritability, Idle, while (59)
Occupation Ameliorates (69)

Work, Desire for Mental (95)

"Occupation Ameliorates" refers to someone who feels much better when they work. The opposite idea is found in "Indolence, Business Aversion to"; "Indifference to Business Affairs"; "Irresolution with Indifference"; "Time, Fritters Away His" and "Work, Aversion to Mental."

The repertory lacks adequate rubrics for psychic experiences. The rubric "Magnetized, Desires to Be" is useful for people who tend to seek out these kind of experiences. Also you can look at "Prophesying," "Clairvoyance," "Dreams, Clairvoyant" (1237), "Dreams, Prophetic," "Dreams, Visionary," and "Death, Presentiment of." The rubrics "Dream, as if in a" and "Unreal, Everything Seems" are related. The former is more of an internal state and the latter is more external.

There are a variety of rubrics pertaining to sexuality. These also can be found under the Female and Male sections of the repertory. Related concepts include:

Fancies, Lascivious (42)
Lasciviousness (61)
Lewdness (62)
Libertinism (62)
Naked, Wants To Be (68)
Nymphomania (68)
Pleasure, Voluptuous Ideas, Only, in (69)
Sexual Excess, Mental Symptoms from (79)
Shameless (79)
Thoughts Intrude and Crowd Around Each Other, Sexual (87)

"Nymphomania" is about uncontrollable sexual desire in women. Some repertories (not Kent's) contain the rubric "Satyriasis" which is the same feeling in men. "Lewdness" and "Lasciviousness" are about an internal lustful state, whereas "Libertinism" is more about unrestrained sexual behavior. "Shamelessness" is a more general state and encompasses behaviors other than sexual behavior. Male sexuality is poorly represented in the *Repertory*.

"Selfishness" and "Egotism" are related. "Selfishness" is more about how one treats others, whereas "Egotism" is more about the attitude that one has about oneself.

"Weeping," "Complaining," and "Lamenting" are related. "Lamenting" is a deeper state and has a sound component associated with it (keening, wailing, or moaning).

"Introspection," "Meditation," "Sits Quietly," "Brooding," "Talk, Indisposed to," "Quiet Disposition," "Secretive," and "Absorbed" are all related concepts. The opposite idea can be found in "Hurried," "Impetuous," "Rashness," "Impatience," and "Time Passes Too Slowly."

Important Rubrics

There are a number of rubrics that come up frequently in prescribing. "Loquacity" refers to much talking or being garrulous. "Fastidious" refers to being overly neat. Related concepts include "Conscientious About Trifles," "Carefulness" and "Rest, Cannot When Things are Not in Their Proper Place." "Forsaken" is a feeling that comes up frequently. This comes up when someone feels abandoned or bereft. Paranoia can be found under the rubric "Suspiciousness." Shyness is found under "Timidity." Anorexia can be found under "Eat, Refuses to." An important part of the Mind section is found under "Sensitivity." In this section you will find "Sensitivity to Noise," "Sensitivity to Light," and "Sensitivity to Music." Sighing is found in the Mind section and not in the Respiratory section. Stubborness is found under "Obstinacy." The desire to be alone is found under "Company, Aversion to." Speech is found in the Mind section, although many of the rubrics related to speech are also found in the Mouth section.

Confusing Terms

Some of the language in the *Repertory* is archaic and confusing. A homeopathic dictionary can be quite helpful in sorting out this terminology (see *A Dictionary of Homeopathic Medical Terminology*, by Jay Yasgur).

"Mania a potu" refers to delirium tremens or d.t.'s. This is a state related to alcohol withdrawal. "Dipsomania" is a term that is synonymous with alcoholism. "Aphasia" refers to impairment or losing the ability to communicate through speech or written language. "Ennui" is defined as boredom or weariness and discontent. "Hydrophobia" is a fear of water. "Somnambulism" is sleep-walking. "Kleptomania" is the compulsion to repeatedly steal.

Delusion Section/Dream Section

The largest rubric in the Mind section is "Delusions." "Delusions" refers to beliefs or feelings that are fixed and false. For many years this section was little used and reserved only for individuals who were more severely mentally ill. Rajan Sankaran has recently opened up this section to more liberal interpretation and much greater usage. He feels that for some individuals there are core delusions from which all of their symptoms spring, and that if we can understand these core delusions, we deepen our understanding of that individual. In the *Spirit of Homeopathy*, he states:

> Delusions are feelings which are not fully based on facts, but they are feelings nevertheless. The difference between delusions and feelings is that delusions are exaggerated, more fixed and often expressed in terms of images.

Delusions can provide living images, which give important clues to the heart of a homeopathic case and a homeopathic remedy.

Sankaran has similarly focused on the usage of the Dream section. This rubric lies in the Sleep section in Kent's repertory, although in many of the more modern repertories it has been placed in the Mind section. He sees dreams as being very close to delusions, representing the core states or essence of an individual (see Lesson Ten). Dreams represent uncompensated material (our true underlying feelings) untainted by our defenses and our need to appear to the outside world other than who we truly are.

Here is an example: A forty-five-year-old woman complains that people can see into her innermost soul. She states she has spent much of her life trying to hide from others to protect herself but could not escape from this. The rubric that I used in this case was "Delusions, Glass, That She is Made of" (26). This is a core delusion of the remedy *Thuja occidentalis,* which acted curatively.

Another example is a young man who is extremely proud and haughty. He talks about looking down on others all the time, and how they are beneath him. The rubric was "Delusions, Small, Things Appear" (p. 32). The remedy was *Platina metalicum,* which again worked curatively.

Studying Materia Medica Through the Repertory

A useful way of studying materia medica is to study all of the rubrics in the repertory that are associated with a particular remedy. There have been several books published which do this for the Mind section of the repertory (*The Complete Materia Medica of the Mind,* by Heli Retzek; *New Comprehensive Materia Medica of the Mind,* by H.L. Chitkara). Studying the materia medica in this way gives a mental/emotional picture for each remedy.

Notes for Lesson Five

Quiz for Lesson Five

Find the appropriate rubric and page number for the following:

1. I am an alcoholic.
2. I am very sensitive to noise. Even the sound of distant church bells bothers me.
3. My brother is extraordinarily shy.
4. My friends tell me that I am the neatest person that they know. I am always cleaning and keep my kitchen spotless.
5. My wife is so paranoid that she doesn't trust anyone.
6. I am a workaholic.
7. My husband is the most detail-focused person that I know.
8. I really love it when I am complimented on my appearance.
9. Whenever my son gets sick, he cannot stand to be touched by anyone.
10. I am always terrified that something bad is about to happen.
11. I get angry right before lunch every day.
12. My son is behaving strangely and engaging in odd behavior.
13. When I get these feelings of depression, it is hard for me to breathe.
14. When I walk into my own house, it is as though I don't recognize anything.
15. I've been thinking about shooting myself with a gun.
16. A young man suffers from tremendous guilt. He states "I feel like I am always being punished for what I have done, especially by God."
17. I always feel terribly guilty.
18. He can never make up his mind. First he wants one thing and then he wants another.
19. He has a history of passing out when he gets very angry.
20. She talks so quickly that I have difficulty following her.

Generalities Section of Kent's Repertory

What Are Generalities?

The Generalities section is found at the end of Kent's *Repertory*. Along with the Mind section, this is one of the most important sections of the *Repertory*. Generalities are symptoms that are true of the whole person rather than of a particular part of the body. They are symptoms of which we can say "I" instead of "My." I may be a chilly person (found in Generalities, p. 1366), but my left leg is what hurts (a particular symptom found in Extremities, p. 1043). Symptoms of the whole are usually more important than symptoms of a particular part. Take a few minutes to read through the Generalities section, pp. 1341–1423.

Time Modalities

The Generalities section begins with time aggravations. "Morning" refers to six to nine a.m., "Forenoon" from ten a.m. until noon, "Afternoon" is one p.m. to five p.m., "Evening" six p.m. to nine p.m., and "Night" nine p.m. until five a.m. Certain remedies are well known for specific time aggravations, although there are many other remedies listed in the Repertory for these time aggravations. These include:

7 a.m. *(Eupatorium perfoliatum)*
9 a.m. *(Chamomilla)*
10 a.m. *(Natrum muriaticum)*
11 a.m. *(Sulphur)*
Noon *(Argentum metallicum)*
2 p.m. *(Pulsatilla nigrans)*
3 p.m. *(Belladonna)*
3–5 p.m. or 4–6 p.m. *(Sepia)*
4 p.m. or 4–8 p.m. *(Lycopodium clavatum)*
Better evening *(Aurum metallicum and Medorrhinum)*
Twilight *(Pulsatilla nigrans and Phosphorous)*
9 p.m. *(Bryonia alba)*
Sunset to sunrise *(Syphilinum)*
11 p.m. *(Cactus grandiflora)*
Better at midnight *(Lycopodium clavatum)*
1 a.m. *(Arsenicum album)*

2–4 a.m. (*Kali carbonicum*)

3 a.m. (*Kali nitricum*)

4 a.m. (*Nux vomica and Carcinosin*) [Note that Carcinosin is not in Kent's Repertory]

5 a.m. (*Podophyllum and Kali iodatum*)

There is a another rubric called "Periodicity." This means any symptoms that tend to recur in a periodic way, whether it be daily, weekly, monthly, or annually. There is also a separate listing for "Breakfast, after" (1346).

Temperature

Chilliness is best found in the rubric "Heat, Lack of Vital" (1366). Other related rubrics are "Cold, Becoming" (1349), "Cold in General Aggravates" (1348), "Uncovering Aggravates" (1410), and "Undressing Aggravates" (1410). There is a Chill section of the *Repertory*. This relates more to infections with chills and fevers rather to feeling cold.

Heat intolerance is best found in the rubric "Heated, on Becoming" (1367). Other related rubrics are "Warm Aggravates" (1412), "Weakness, Worse Heat" (1417), "Sun Aggravates" (1404), and "Summer Aggravates" (1404). There is also a Fever section of the *Repertory* which again is more related to infections. Hot flushes (i.e., menopausal hot flushes) are found under "Heat, Flushes of."

Weather

There are a variety of weather aggravations. There is a section for "Air" (1343), which contains "Open Air, Ameliorates" and "Open Air, Aggravates." Also, you will find here "Air, Seashore Aggravates" and "Air, Seashore Ameliorates." This is the best rubric for people who are better or worse at the seashore. Other weather rubrics include:

Autumn (1345)

Change of Temperature (1347)

Change of Weather (1347)

Clear Weather (1348)

Cloudy Weather (1348)

Cold Dry Weather (1349)

Cold Wet Weather (1350)

Dry Weather (1357)

Foggy Weather (1362)

Moonlight (1374)

Snowy Air (1402)

Spring (1403)
Storm Approach (1403)
Summer (1404)
Sun (1404)
Vaults=Basements [Cold and damp] (1411)
Warm Wet Weather (1413)
Wet Weather (1421)
Wind (1422)
Windy Stormy Weather (1422)
Winter (1422)

Modalities

There are separate sections for "Air" (1343) and "Wind" (1422). "Drafts" are found under the Air section, along with "Desire for" and "Aversion to" Open Air.

Desire and aversion for alcohol are found in the Stomach section. Those who are generally worse from alcohol can be found in the rubric "Alcoholic Stimulants" (1344). Related rubrics include "Intoxication" (1369), "Reveling From Night" (1397) and "Wine" (1422).

There are a number of rubrics in the *Repertory* pertaining to clothing. Perhaps the most useful is "Clothing, Intolerance of" (1348). This idea can also be found in the section "External Throat, Clothing Aggravates" (471) and in the section "Abdomen, Clothing Sensitive to" (541). Related rubrics are "Undressing Aggravates" (1410) and "Uncovering Aggravates" (1410).

There are a variety of body functions listed in the Generalities section. These include:

Loss of Fluids [i.e., Extended diarrhea or hemorrhage] (1371)
Menses (1373)
Perspiration (1391)
Sleep (1401)
Vomiting (1411)
Waking (1411)

Again, note that these rubrics refer to general aggravations at the time of these activities.

There are separate listings for body types. These include:

Dwarfism (1357)
Lean (1370)
Nursing Children (1376)
Obesity (1376)

Old People (1376)
Stoop Shouldered (1403)

A small but useful rubric is "Contradictory and Alternating States" (1351). This refers to conditions that rapidly change from one polarity to another in a confusing and unpredictable manner. An example would be a young man who complains of intense coldness in his hands alternating with severe heat. The condition changes so rapidly that at times he complains of both simultaneously.

"Faintness" (1358) is a useful rubric in the Generalities section. This should be distinguished from "Vertigo," which has its own section. Faintness is more nonspecific and nonlocalizing. It is often described as a complaint of lightheadedness, dizziness, giddiness, floating, swaying, or disorientation. Generally it is not associated with any specific accompanying signs. Vertigo is the illusion of movement or rotation of the environment about someone. It can also be the illusion of rotation, tilting, or oscillation of the environment. It is often associated with nausea or vomiting and balance problems.

There are a variety of rubrics relating to food. These include:

Eating (1357)
Fasting [this is a useful rubric to describe hypoglycemia] (1361)
Food (1362)
Hunger from (1367)
Starving (1403)
Tobacco Aggravates (1407)

The Food section refers to feeling generally worse from eating certain foods. Food desires and aversions are found in the Stomach section.

Motions of the body include:

Chorea [dance-like writhing movements] (1347)
Convulsions [seizures] (1351)
Convulsive Movements (1356)
Jerking (1369)
Quivering (1397)
Shuddering Nervous (1400)
Trembling (1407)
Twitching (1409)

There is also a separate rubric for Parkinson's Disease ("Paralysis agitans").

Long-term effects of exposure to various toxins and poisons are found in the Generalities section. Larger sections for these problems can be found in Boericke's

Pocket Manual of Homeopathic Materia Medica with Repertory and Murphy's *Homeopathic Medical Repertory.* These include:

Arsenical (1345)
China (1347)
Coal Gas (1348)
Copper (1356)
Iron (1369)
Lead (1370)
Mercury (1374)
Quinine (1397)
Silica (1401)
Smoke (1402)
Sulphur (1404)

Aggravations related to position include:

Change of Position (1347)
Kneeling (1370)
Lying (1371)
Rising (1397)
Sitting (1401)
Standing (1403)
Stretching (1403)

"Pulse" (1393) is a fairly extensive section that describes various types of pulses. These include irregular, hard, imperceptible, frequent, fluttering, slow, and weak. There are a variety of purposeful activities that cause aggravations. These include:

Ascending (1345)
Bathing (1345)
Descending (1356)
Exertion (1358)
Jarring (1369)
Lifting (1371)
Motion (1374)
Playing Piano [use this also for repetitive typing on the computer] (1390)
Riding [can use the subrubric for motion sickness] (1397)
Rising (1397)
Rubbing (1398)
Running (1398)
Stretching (1403)

Touching (1407)

Walking (1411)

Motion sickness can also be found in the Stomach section under "Nausea, Riding in a Carriage" (509).

Much of the Generalities section is taken up with sensations of the body. These include:

Analgesia [painlessness of something normally painful] (1345)

Ball (1345)

Bubbling (1346)

Caged (1346)

Coat of Skin Drawn Over Inner Parts (1348)

Constriction (1350)

Flabby (1361)

Foreign Bodies or Grains of Sand Were Under the Skin (1364)

Formification [creeping, crawling sensation on skin like insects crawling on it] (1364)

Frail (1365)

Full (1365)

Hair Sensation (1365)

Hard Bed (1365)

Heaviness (1367)

Knotted (1370)

Numbness [loss of all sensation] (1375)

Orgasm of Blood [sudden rush of blood to the affected part-adrenaline rush like feeling] (1376),

Painlessness of Complaints Usually Painful [see also analgesia] (1390)

Plug (1391)

Prickling (1392)

Pulsation (1392)

Sensitiveness (1398)

Shocks (1399)

Shot Rolling Through Arteries (1400)

Smaller (1402)

Stagnated as if Blood (1403)

Streaming of Blood (1403)

Strength (1403)

Swollen (1406)

Tension (1406)

Threads (1407)

Trickling Like Drops (1409)

Water Dashing Against Inner Parts (1413)
Wave Like (1413)
Worms Under the Skin Sensation (1422)

Sexual aggravations are found in a variety of locations in the Generalities section. These include "Coition" [sexual intercourse] (1348), "Emissions Aggravate" (1358), "Onanism" [sexual withdrawal before intercourse] (1376) and "Sexual Excesses" (1399). Some of these ideas can also be found in the Genitalia sections.

An important rubric is "Sides" (1400). This is where you would look for a condition where someone only had symptoms on one side of their body. Subrubrics here include "One Side," "Alternating Sides," "Crosswise," "Right" and "Left."

"Vaccination" (1410) refers to ailments following a vaccination. This condition is also called vaccinosis. Kent's *Repertory* refers only to the smallpox vaccination, as no other vaccinations were available at the time of writing. In more modern repertories, this has been expanded to include other vaccinations.

"Bathing" (1345) is a useful rubric. The subrubrics include "Bathing, Dread Of" (1345) and "Bathing Ameliorates" (1345). There is a separate listing for "Uncleanliness Aggravates" (1410).

There are a variety of rubrics that touch on the idea of fatigue. These include:

Collapse (1350)
Fainting (1358)
Lassitude (1370)
Reaction, Lack of [inability of the body to muster a defense against disease] (1397)
Sluggishness of the Body (1402)
Weakness (1413)
Weariness (1421)

These are useful rubrics to consider for Chronic Fatigue Syndrome.

Diseases

There are a variety of diseases that are included in the Generalities section. Most of the diseases in the *Repertory* are found here. There only only a few diseases listed. Remedies are generally prescribed on symptoms and not on specific diseases. Many of the well known diseases of today were not well known or understood at the time of the writing of the repertory. Specific diseases found here include:

Abscess [a collection of pus in a circumscribed cavity] (1343)
Anemia [deficiency of blood constituents] (1344)
Apoplexy [stroke] (1345)

Cancerous Affections [see also "Tumors" and "Ulcers, Cancerous"] (1346)

Caries of Bones [dental cavities or pockets of degeneration of bones] (1346)

Catalepsy [trance-like state with rigidity of limbs that remain in the same position for a long period of time, catatonia] (1347)

Chlorosis [iron-deficiency anemia] (1347)

Cold, Tendency to Take [recurrent upper respiratory infections] (1349)

Contracture/Strictures After Inflammation [the constriction of tissue after an inflammation] (1351)

Convulsions [seizures] (1351)

Cyanosis [blue discoloration of the body resulting from lack of oxygenation to the tissues: see "Face, discoloration, blueness"] (1356)

Dropsy [edema/swelling: see also "Extremities, Swelling, Lower Limbs, Dropsical"] (1356)

Emaciation [malnourished or underweight] (1357)

Exostoses [bony hard overgrowths] (1358)

Glanders [disease of horses with swollen lymph nodes and ulceration] (1365)

Gonorrhea Suppressed (1365)

Hemorrhage [bleeding] (1365)

Leukemia [cancerous disease of the white blood cells] (1370)

Measles After [see "Fever, Exanthematic, Measles"] (1373)

Necrosis of Bones [destruction of bony tissue] (1375)

Obesity (1376)

Paralysis Agitans [Parkinson's disease] (1390)

Polypus [growth extending from a mucous membrane] (1391)

Scarlet Fever [see "Fever, Exanthematic, Scarlatina"] (1398)

Scurvy [vitamin C deficiency] (1398)

Septicemia [infection of the blood] (1399)

Sycosis (1406)

Syphilis (1406)

Thrombosis [blood clot] (1407)

Ulcers (1410)

Varicose Veins (1410)

Diabetes is not listed in the Generalities section, but can be found under "Urine Sugar" (691). Thyroid disease and goiters are found in "External Neck, Goiter" (471). Malaria is found in the Fever section under "Remittent" and in the Chill section under "Quartan," "Quotidian," or "Tertian." Meningitis (inflammation of the membranes surrounding the brain and spinal cord) is found under "Fever, Cerebrospinal" (1282) or "Head, Inflammation, Meningitis" (128). Parasites are located in the Rectum section under "Worms" (634). The Generalities section contains rubrics for Sycosis and Syphilis. There is no specific rubric for Psora. Tuberculosis is found under "Chest, Phthisis" (878).

A variety of injuries are found throughout the *Repertory,* many of which lie in the Generalities section. These include:

> Injuries (1368)
> Burns (1346)
> Shocks from Injury (1399)
> Slow Repair of Bones (1402)
> Bites of Poisonous Animals (1422)
> Wounds (1422)

Sunstroke can be found in the Head section under "Sunstroke" (231). Head injuries can be found in the Head section under "Concussion" (109) or "Injuries" (128). Stings of insects can be found in the Skin section under "Stings of Insects" (1331). There is also a listing in the Extremities section for "Injuries" (1019).

Other Confusing Rubrics

"Puerperal Convulsions" (1353) refers to convulsions of pregnancy. "Atrophy" (1345) means a wasting or shrinkage of tissue. "Clonic Convulsions" (1352) are seizures characterized by an alternating contraction and release of the muscles. "Tonic Convulsions" (1355) are more of a steady contracted state. "Extensor Muscles" (1353) refer to muscles that tend to straighten or extend a part of the body. "Fistulae" (1361) are abnormal passages between a body cavity and the surface or between two body cavities. "Indurations" (1367) are hardenings of tissue. "Excessive Physical Irritability" (1369) refers to a nervous system that is excessively sensitive and wound up. "Magnetism Ameliorates" (1373) is about individuals who feel better when they are hypnotized or placed in a trance state. "Metastasis" (1374) refers to symptoms that jump from one part of the body to another. The symptoms are not necessarily related to each other. An example would be the remedy *Abrotanum,* which has rheumatic arthritis following diarrhea. "Plethora" (1391) is an excess of any bodily fluid, although most often relates to excess of blood in a particular area. This often manifests as flushing of the skin, redness, and heat.

Notes for Lesson Six

Quiz for Lesson Six

Find the best rubric and page number in the *Repertory* for each symptom:

1. All my symptoms occur only on the left side of my body.
2. I feel better when I exercise.
3. Whenever I have dental work, I pass out from the pain.
4. All my pains appear and disappear suddenly.
5. Ever since I had a shot of morphine for my last migraine headache, I have felt terrible. I never recovered.
6. I feel much worse before every period.
7. All the glands in my body feel tremendously sore.
8. My doctor tells me that I have iron-deficiency anemia.
9. I feel worse every time I climb stairs.
10. Ever since menopause, I have been having these severe hot flashes.
11. I absolutely hate to wash. It makes me afraid.
12. My husband feels worse every Fall.
13. My husband tells me that I am the chilliest person that he knows.
14. I feel much better at the ocean.
15. I only feel better after midnight.
16. My daughter feels much better every time she smokes.
17. My father has Parkinson's Disease.
18. I have a strong family history of tuberculosis that dates back for many generations.
19. I feel trapped. It is as if everyone has these strings around me that are pulling tighter and tighter.
20. My epileptic convulsions seem to come regularly if I am about to meet someone or go on a date, or if ever I am looking forward to something or even if I am a little nervous.

Vertigo Through Mouth Sections of Kent's Repertory

General Comments

What follows is a brief exploration of each of the remaining sections of the *Repertory*. Take a few minutes to review each section before reading the comments listed below. I will focus on the more commonly used rubrics in each section that are clinically useful, as well as help you to understand the meaning of any unusual rubrics. You will also find a glossary of repertory terminology in Appendix H.

If you are new to anatomy, the terminology can be quite confusing. *The Dictionary of Homeopathic Medical Terminology,* by Jay Yasgur, is quite helpful, along with a pictorial guide such as *Grant's Atlas of Anatomy* by James Anderson, M.D.

Certain important general concepts are common to almost every section. These include Coldness, Discoloration, Eruptions, Heat, Inflammation, Itching, Motion, Numbness, Pain, Perspiration, Sensitive, Stiffness, and Swelling. Warts are listed at times under "Warts" and at times under "Condylomata." Menopause is sometimes referred to as "Menopause" and at other times as "Climaxis."

Anterior refers to being in the front or being situated before something else. Posterior is behind or at the back. Dorsal also refers to the back, whereas ventral refers to the front.

Vertigo

Vertigo was felt to be so important that it has its own section. Vertigo, or dizziness, refers to an abnormal sensation of motion, either of oneself or of external objects. It is often associated with a tendency to fall. It is often accompanied by nausea or vomiting. It usually represents a problem in the vestibular apparatus of the inner ear, although it can originate from deeper in the brain. This should be distinguished from "Fainting" in the Generalities section, which is a more general state often resulting from a lack of blood supply to the brain. Fainting is synonymous with light-headedness.

Important Rubrics:

Chronic (98)
Closing Eyes (98)
Concussion from (98)
Continuous (98)

Coughing (98)
Epilepsy (98)
Falling Sensation (99)
Fall, Tendency to [in various directions] (99)
Floating, as if (99)
Headache During (99)
High Places (100)
Injuries of Head after (100)
Looking [in a variety of directions] (100)
Lying (101)
Menses (101)
Mental Exertion (101)
Motion from (101)
Moving the Head (101)
Nausea with (102)
Old People (102)
Pregnancy (102)
Reeling [identical to staggering] (102)
Rising (102)
Standing (104)
Stooping (104)
Sudden (105)
Sunlight and Heat (105)
Turning of the Head (105)
Vision, Obscuration of (105)
Walking (106)

Confusing Terms:

"Diplopia" (98) refers to double vision.

"Syncope" (105) refers to fainting.

"Watching and Loss of Sleep" (106) refers to taking care of someone who is sick and thus staying up all night. This is also referred to in the *Repertory,"*as Night Watching.

Head

The Head section of the Repertory covers from above the eyebrows, over the top of the head (vertex), to the back of the head (occiput). It includes the scalp and excludes the face and neck. "Head, Heat, Flashes of" (122) is useful for the idea of hot flushes. The rubrics "Congestion" (109) and "Sensation of Brain Swelling" (232) are useful for chemical hypersensitivity. The scalp and hair are found here, as well as in the Skin section.

Important Rubrics:

    Asleep, Sensation as if (107)

    Bores Head into Pillow (108)

    Cerebral Hemorrhage (108)

    Coldness (108)

    Cold Air, Sensitive to (109)

    Concussion (109)

    Constriction [subrubric band or hoop is useful] (111)

    Dandruff (114)

    Empty Hollow Sensation (114)

    Eruptions (115)

    Exostoses [bony overgrowth] (117)

    Formication [crawling sensation like insects on the skin (118)

    Fullness (118)

    Hair [subrubric "Falling, Gray Prematurely"] (120)

    Heat (121)

    Heaviness (124)

    Inflammation of the Meninges (128)

    Itching (129)

    Looseness of the Brain Sensation (129)

    Motions [a variety of motions in and of the head] (130)

    Numbness(132)

    Open Fontanelles [the area on the top of a baby's head, commonly referred to as the soft spot] (132)

    Pain (132)

    Perspiration of the Scalp (221)

    Sensitiveness (229)

    Shocks Blows Jerks (230)

    Sunstroke (231)

    Swollen Feeling (232)

    Twitching of Muscles (232)

    Uncovering Aggravates (233)

    Washing Aggravates (234)

    Weakness (234)

Confusing Terms:

    "Cephalhaematoma" (108) is a bloody cyst or tumor of the scalp.

    "Congestion or Hyperaemia" (109) is an increased amount of blood in the head.

    "Hydrocephalus" (128) refers to an accumulation of fluid in the ventricles of the brain causing compression of the brain.

Occiput is the lower back of the head, where the head meets the neck.
Vertex is the top of the head.

Eye

The Eye section covers symptoms related to the eyeball and eyelid but not the eyebrows, which are found in the Face section.

Agglutinated [eyelids stuck together] (235)
Bleeding (235)
Brilliant [sparkling] (235)
Cataract (236)
Chemosis [swelling of the conjunctiva](236)
Close [a multitude of subrubrics pertaining to eye closure](236)
Condylomata [warts] (237)
Discharges (237)
Dryness (238)
Ecchymosis [bruising] (238)
Glaucoma [elevated eye pressure, which can result in blindness] (240)
Heat in (241)
Heaviness (241)
Injected [redness] (244)
Inflammation [you will find conjunctivitis here] (241)
Irritation (244)
Itching (244)
Lachrymation [tears] (245)
Movement [a variety of types of movement] (246)
Open [a multitude of subrubrics pertaining to eye opening] (247)
Pain (248)
Photophobia [intolerance to light] (261)
Protrusion (262)
Pupils [a variety of subrubrics pertaining to pupils] (263)
Redness (264)
Rub, Desire To (265)
Sensitive (265)
Spasms (265)
Staring (265)
Strabismus [lack of parallel vision in the eyes] (266)
Styes (266)
Swollen (267)
Turned [in a variety of directions] (268)
Twitching (269)

Ulceration (269)

Weak (270)

Winking (270)

Confusing Terms

"Arcus Senilis" (247) is a white ring around the cornea found in the elderly.

"Astigmatism" is an unequal curvature of the eye, causing blurred vision (235).

"Atrophy of the Optic Nerve" (235) is wasting of the nerve.

"Canthi" (243) are the corners of the eye, both inner and outer.

"Cataract Reticularis" (236) refers to a netlike cataract.

"Cataract Viridis" (236) is a green cataract.

"Choroid" (243) is the sheath surrounding the eye that carries the blood supply.

"Cortical" (236) refers to originating from the brain vs. originating from the eye itself.

"Esophoria" (239) is a turning of the eye inwards.

"Eversion of Lids" (239) is a tendency for the upper eyelid to flip upwards.,"

"Onyx" (247) is an abscess of the cornea.

"Pannus" (261) refers to a grey membrane covering part, or the entire, cornea. "Photomania" (261) is an intense desire for light.

"Pterygium" (262) is a triangular patch of tissue beginning in the corner of the eye.

"Staphyloma" (265) refers to a bulging of the cornea due to inflammation.

Vision

Vision is a smaller section following Eyes. Note that functionalities like Vision, Hearing, Cough, etc., follow the same format of a related anatomical area, such as Eyes, Ears, and Respiration. Blindness and visual distortions are also found here.

Important rubrics:

Accommodation, Defective [ability of the eyes to adjust to light or distance](271)

Acute (271)

Blurred (271)

Circles (271)

Colors (272)

Dim (275)

Diplopia [double vision] (277)

Distant, Objects Seem (278)

Flickering (278)

Foggy (278)

Hypermetropia [far sightedness] (280)

Illusions[also see delusion section] (280)

Loss of Vision[blindness] (281)

Moving (282)

Myopia [near-sightedness] (283)

Sparks (283)

Spots (284)

Weak (284)

Confusing Terms:

"Hemiopia" (280) is vision on one side.

"Incipient Cataract" (279) refers to a newly emerging cataract.

"Scotoma" (283) is a blind spot.

"Triplopia" (284) is triple vision.

Ear

This section includes the inner and outer ear. Areas on the head directly adjoining the ear are also found here. The largest section is "Ear, Pain" (303). Ear infections can be found under "Ear, Inflammation, Media" (291) and "Ear, Pain, Inside" (307). Sounds that originate from outside the ear are found here. Sounds that originate from within the ear are found in the next section (Hearing).

Important rubrics:

Air, Sensation of In (285)

Boring Fingers In (285)

Catarrh [mucus discharge] (285)

Coldness (285)

Discharges (286)

Discoloration (287)

Dryness (287)

Eruptions (287)

Fullness, Sensation of (289)

Heat (290)

Inflammation (290)

Itching (291)

Noises in [many subrubrics including ringing] (292)

Numbness (302)

Pain (303)

Pulsation (316)
Stopped Sensation (317)
Swelling (318)
Twitching (319)
Ulceration (319)
Wax (320)

Confusing Terms:

"Antitragus" (318) is a cartilage projection of the outer ear.

"Concha" (290) is the outer ear.

"Eustachian Tube" (291) refers to the auditory canal connecting the ear with the throat.

"Mastoid" (313) refers to the area behind the ear, felt as a pointed bone.

"Tympanum" (285) is the ear drum.

Hearing

This is a very small section. Important rubrics include "Acute" (321) and "Impaired" (321). There is a subrubric of "Impaired Lost" (328), which refers to deafness. Another useful subrubric is "Impaired, Catarrh of Eustachian Tube" (322), which refers to hearing loss due to fluid or mucous in the ear *(serous otitis media)*. Illusions of hearing are also found here (321).

Nose

Unlike Hearing and Vision, Smell does not have a separate subsection and is listed under Nose. Many of the rubrics for allergies are found here. The words "Catarrh" (324) and "Coryza" (325) can be used interchangeably, indicating a mucous discharge from the nose, related either to an upper respiratory infection or to an allergic response. The subrubric "Coryza, Annual" (326) is used to describe hay fever. The Odor section is reserved for specific odors, whereas the Smell section is about the ability to smell. "Catarrh, Post Nasal" (325) is the rubric to use for post-nasal drip. This section does not include most of the sinuses, which are found more in the Face and Head sections.

Important rubrics:

Blow, Constant Inclination to (324)
Boring in with Fingers (324)
Catarrh [secretion of mucus caused by inflammation of mucus membrane related to irritants] (324)
Coldness (325)
Coryza [mucus discharge related to a cold] (325)

Discharge (329)
Discoloration (334)
Dryness (334)
Epistaxis [nose bleeds] (335)
Fullness, Sense of (338)
Heat (338)
Inflammation (339)
Itching (339)
Numbness (340)
Obstruction (340)
Odors (341)
Pain (343)
Picking Nose (348)
Smell (349)
Sneezing (350)
Snuffles (351)
Swelling (352)
Ulcers (353)
Warts (352)

Confusing Terms:
"Dorsum" (347) refers to the back of the nose.
"Ozaena" (343) is a fetid/foul nasal discharge, often accompanied by
   ulceration.
"Posterior nares" (335) are the nasal cavities in the back of the nose.
"Root" (346) is the top of the nose.
"Septum" (345) is the wall separating the two nasal cavities.
"Wings" (334) refers to the sides of the nose.

Face

The Face section of the *Repertory* covers from below the eyebrows to the neck, excluding the eyes, ears, mouth, and nose. It includes the outer surface of the mouth. The sinuses are not well represented in Kent's *Repertory*. Related sinus rubrics include "Catarrhal Headache" (137), "Face, Pain, Extending to Cheek" (383), "Face, Pain, Eye, Below" (383), "Face, Pain, Sore Bruised" (387), "Nose, Catarrh, Extending to Frontal Sinuses" (325) and "Head, Pain, Forehead, Middle Frontal Sinuses from Chronic Coryza" (161). Acne is found under "Face, Eruptions, Acne" (366). The eyelids are in the Face section and anything around the nose is in the Face section. Cold sores can be found under "Face, Eruptions, Herpetic, Lips" (369). Facial expressions are found here (374) and not in the Mind section.

Useful rubrics:

Bloated (355)

Chapped Lips (356)

Clenched Jaw [see also teeth section] (356)

Coldness (356)

Convulsions (357)

Cracked Lips (357)

Cracking in Jaw when Chewing [good rubric for TMJ] (357)

Discoloration (357)

Distortion (364)

Dryness (364)

Eruptions (365)

Erysipelas [superficial cellulitis or skin infection caused by Beta-
hemolytic Streptococcus] (373)

Expression [a multitude of facial expressions] (374)

Freckles (375)

Heat (375)

Inflammation (378)

Itching (378)

Numbness (379)

Pain (379)

Paralysis (390)

Perspiration (390)

Sensitive (391)

Stiffness (392)

Swelling (392)

Tension of Skin [useful for scleroderma] (394)

Twitching (395)

Ulcers (395)

Warts (396)

Confusing Terms:

"Acne Rosacea" (366) is a type of acne associated with the breakdown of
capillaries of the skin, causing dark red blotches.

"Comedones" (367) are blackheads.

"Hippocratic" (378) refers to sunken and prematurely old-looking.

"Impetigo" (369) is a contagious skin disease, mostly of children, characterized by pustular skin eruptions on the face.

"Malar Bone" (394) is the cheek-bone or zygoma.

"Masseter Muscle" (394) is the muscle in the jaw used for chewing.

"Risus Sardonicus" (391) is a fixed grin caused by spasms around the
mouth.

"Sordes on the Lips" (392) relates to the black crust found on the lips during typhoid fever.

"Zygoma" (368) is the cheek bone.

Mouth

The mucous membranes of the mouth are found here. Taste is found within the Mouth section and does not follow the same format as the Vision section or Hearing section. There is a speech section in Mouth that refers to the qualities of speech. You can also find Speech in the Mind section (81). There is a great deal of overlap between these two sections. Stuttering is found in the Mouth section. Chancre sores can be found under "Mouth, Aphthae" (397). The teeth are found in a separate section that follows.

Important rubrics:

Abscess, Gums (397)
Tongue Adheres to Roof of Mouth (397)
Aphthae [chancre sores] (397)
Biting (397)
Bleeding (397)
Coldness (399)
Cold Breath (399)
Cracked (399)
Gums Detached from Teeth (399)
Discoloration (400)
Dryness (403)
Heat (405)
Inflammation (406)
Itching (406)
Motion (407)
Mucus (407)
Mucous Membrane (408)
Numbness (408)
Odor [various odors] (409)
Open (409)
Pain (410)
Paralysis (415)
Protruded (415)
Saliva [characteristics of the saliva] (416)
Salivation (417)
Sensitive (418)
Speech (419)

Swelling (420)
Taste (421)
Trembling (427)
Ulcers (428)
Vesicles (429)

Confusing Terms:

"Cancrum Oris" (398) is a severe and often fatal disease of children, producing a gangrenous ulceration of the mucous membranes of the mouth.

"Epulis" (404) is a small tumor of the gum.

"Fraenum" (429) is the fold of tissue that connects the tongue to the bottom of the mouth.

"Papillae" (406) are small nipplelike projections at the root of the tongue.

"Ranula" (416) is an obstruction of the sublingual gland duct by a cystic tumor on the bottom of the mouth.

"Root" (410) is the base or back of the tongue.

"Scorbutic Gums" (418) refer to spongy bleeding gums related to Vitamin C deficiency.

"Sordes" (419) are the black crusts found in the mouth during typhoid fever.

"Stomacace" (420) is an ulcerative inflammation of the mouth.

"Velum" (406) is the extension at the back of the hard palate that separates the mouth from the pharynx.

Notes for Lesson Seven

Quiz for Lesson Seven

Choose the best rubric and page number for the following:

1. I have difficulty adjusting to the bright lights from oncoming cars when I am driving at night.
2. My son's ears get bright red every evening.
3. I have dizziness that makes me fall to the right side.
4. I keep getting warts around my mouth.
5. Ever since my wife insulted me in front of my colleagues, I haven't been able to hear as well.
6. My son drools on his pillow every night when he sleeps.
7. My wife is sensitive to the smell of any cooking.
8. The baby is always sucking its fingers.
9. My daughter's head perspires a great deal during sleep.
10. I always get a bad headache when I eat too much.
11. When I wake up in the morning it seems like everything is flickering.
12. It looks as though there is a green film in front of my eyes.
13. I get a headache at the top of my head that feels like a nail being driven in. This occurs every night at 3 a.m.
14. Whenever I first get my migraine headaches, I cannot see.
15. I have conjunctivitis.
16. I often have the feeling of spider webs brushing my face.
17. I keep getting these chancre sores on the tip of my tongue.
18. I get nosebleeds instead of having my period.
19. I get this strange metallic taste in my mouth.
20. I think that I am going bald.

Teeth Through Respiration

Teeth

Teeth grinding, or bruxism, is found under "Teeth, Grinding, Sleep During" (432). Teething problem's of children can be found under "Teeth, Dentition, Difficult" (431) or "Teeth, Dentition, Slow" (431). The majority of this section is taken up with "Teeth, Pain."

Important rubrics:

Caries, Decayed (431)
Clinch Together Constant Inclination [see "Bite Together, Desire To"] (431)
Coldness (431)
Dentition (431)
Discolored (431)
Grinding (432)
Looseness Of (432)
Nerves, Injuries to Dental Nerves (433)
Pain (433)
Sensitive (446)
Wisdom Teeth, Ailments from Eruption of (447)

Confusing Terms:

"Canines" (433) are the pointed teeth situated next to the incisors.
"Incisors" (433) are the four front teeth used for cutting.
"Masticating, from" (437) refers to chewing.
"Malar Bone" (442) refers to the cheekbone.
"Molars" (433) are teeth that have a broad biting surface adapted to grinding; they are on each side of both the upper and lower jaw.
"Zygoma" (445) also refers to the cheek bone.

Throat

The esophagus, pharynx, tonsils, and uvula are found here. Symptoms related to voice and coughing are listed in a separate section (Larynx and Trachea).

Important rubrics:

Choking (448)
Coldness (449)
Discoloration (450)
Dryness (450)
Enlargement of Tonsils (451)
Foreign Body Sensation (452)
Fullness (452)
Hawk, Disposition to (452)
Heat (453)
Inflammation (453)
Irritation (454)
Itching (454)
Lump Sensation (454)
Mucus (456)
Numbness (458)
Pain [many useful rubrics here for sore throats] (458)
Paralysis (465)
Roughness (465)
Scraping [clearing throat] (466)
Sensitive (466)
Spasms (467)
Suppuration of Tonsils [pus] (467)
Swallow, Constant Disposition To (467)
Swallowing Difficult (467)
Swelling (469)
Tension (469)
Ulcers (470)

Confusing Terms:

"Aphthae" (448) are chancre sores.

"Drawn from Posterior Nares" (456) means coming from the back of the nose [see also "Catarrh, Post Nasal"].

"Fauces" (456) is another name for the sides of the throat.

"Uvula" (450) is a small fleshy conical membrane of tissue projecting downward from the middle of the upper soft palate in the mouth.

External Throat

This is a very small section. It includes the anterior sections of the external neck. The posterior of the neck is found in the Back section. Goiter is found here.

Hyperthyroidism is best found in "Goitre, Exophthalmic" [causing protrusion of the eyes] (472). There is no good rubric for hypothyroidism in this repertory. Swollen lymph nodes are found under either "Swelling, Cervical Glands" (473) or "Pain, Cervical Glands" (472). "Clothing Aggravates" (471) is also found here.

Important rubrics:

> Abscess (471)
> Clothing Aggravates (471)
> Coldness (471)
> Constriction (471)
> Discoloration (471)
> Eruption (471)
> Goitre (471)
> Induration of the Glands (472)
> Itching (472)
> Pain (472)
> Perspiration (474)
> Pulsation (474)
> Stiffness (474)
> Swelling (474)
> Tension (474)
> Uncovering Throat Aggravates (475)

Confusing Terms:

> "Cervical Glands" (473) are lymph nodes or glands of the neck.
> "Torticollis" (475) is a spasmodic contraction of the muscles of the neck, causing the head to be drawn to one side.

Stomach

Food cravings (483) and aversions (480) are found in this section. In more modern repertories these rubrics may be placed in the Generalities section. Food aggravations, however, are found in the Generalities section. Spicy foods can be found under "Desires, Highly Seasoned" (485). Pica can be found under "Desires, Indigestibles" (485). Thirst and appetite are also located here. Nausea and Vomiting are located in this section and not under abdomen. "Nausea, Pregnancy of" (509) is found here. Motion sickness can be found under "Nausea, Riding in a Carriage" or "Nausea, Seasickness" (509). Swelling or bloating is found under "Distension" (487).

Important rubrics:

> Anxiety (476)

Appetite (476)
Aversions (480)
Clothing Disturbs (482)
Coldness (482)
Constriction (483)
Disordered (486)
Distension (487)
Emptiness (487)
Eructations [belching] (489)
Fullness (498)
Gagging (499)
Gurgling (499)
Heartburn (499)
Heat (500)
Heaviness (501)
Hiccough (501)
Indigestion (503)
Inflammation (503)
Nausea (504)
Pain (511)
Retching [dry heaves] (525)
Tension (527)
Thirst (527)
Thirstless (530)
Ulcers (531)
Vomiting (531)

Confusing Terms:

"Farinaceous Foods" (480) refer to starchy food such as pasta, bread, and grains.

"Retraction Sense of" (526) refers to a pulling back of the abdomen.

"Waterbrash" (497) is a watery acid wash from the stomach. This is a useful rubric for acid reflux.

Abdomen

There are nine anatomical divisions of the abdomen. The upper left quadrant is the left hypochondriac, the upper central quadrant is the epigastric, the upper right quadrant is the right hypochondriac, the central quadrant is the umbilical, the left central quadrant is the left lumbar (side), the right central quadrant is the right lumbar (side), the left lower quadrant is the left iliac (inguinal), the lower central quadrant is the hypogastric, and the lower right quadrant is the right iliac (inguinal). See Appendix J for a visual representation of these divisions.

Important rubrics:

Anxiety in (541)

Cirrhosis of Liver [chronic destruction of the liver resulting in liver failure] (541)

Clothing, Sensitive to (541)

Coldness (542)

Constriction (542)

Discoloration (544)

Distension (544)

Dropsy Ascites [accumulation of fluids] (546)

Emptiness (546)

Enlarged [various organs] (546)

Eruptions (547)

Flatulence (547)

Fullness Sensation (549)

Gurgling (550)

Heat (551)

Hernia (552)

Inflammation (552)

Itching (553)

Liver and Region of (553)

Movements in (554)

Pain (554)

Perspiration (599)

Retraction (600)

Rumbling (600)

Swelling (602)

Tension (603)

Ulcers (605)

Confusing Terms:

"Aneurism" (541) is a dilation of an artery.

"Ilio Caecal" (565) is the end of the large intestine in the lower right quadrant.

"Ilium" (564) is the flank area or the upper portion of the hip bone.

"Intussusception" (553) is a telescoping of one section of the intestine into another section.

"Pendulous Abdomen" (599) refers to hanging loosely.

"Tabes Mesenterica" (603) refers to tuberculosis with enlarged lymph nodes.

"Tympanitic" (545) means distended with a hyperresonant sound, like a drum.

"Typhlitis" (553) refers to appendicitis.

Rectum

This section refers to the functioning of the rectum itself. The Rectum section contains "Constipation," and "Diarrhea." Constipation can be found under "Constipation" as well as under "Inactivity of the Rectum." Hemorrhoids can be found here. This is also where you find "Worms" (634).

Important rubrics:

Coldness (606)
Condylomata [warts] (606)
Constipation (606)
Constriction (608)
Diarrhea (609)
Dysentery [infectious disease causing diarrhea] (616)
Eruptions (616)
Fissure (617)
Fistula (617)
Flatus (617)
Formification [creeping, crawling sensation, like insects crawling] (618)
Haemorrhage (619)
Haemorrhoids (619)
Heat (621)
Involuntary Stool (621)
Itching (622)
Lump Sensation (623)
Pain (623)
Paralysis (631)
Polypi (631)
Prolapsus (631)
Stricture (632)
Swelling (632)
Urging Desire (633)
Worms (634)

Confusing Terms:

"Ascarides" (634) and "Lumbricoides" (635) are roundworms.

"Cholera" (606) is a bacterial infection causing severe diarrhea, vomiting, and wasting.

"Perineum" (616) is the space in front of the rectum.

"Portal Stasis" (608) is a reduced flow of blood through the liver.

"Taeniae" (635) are tapeworms.

"Tenesmus" (630) are involuntary contractions.

Stool

The Stool section is about the qualities of the stool itself. The functioning of the rectum is found in the Rectum section.

Important rubrics:

Black (635)

Bloody (635)

Copious (636)

Frequent (637)

Green (637)

Hard (638)

Large (638)

Lienteric [undigested food present] (638)

Mucous (639)

Odor (640)

Pasty (641)

Scanty (641)

Soft (641)

Thin (642)

Watery (643)

White (644)

Yellow (644)

Urinary Organs (Bladder, Kidneys, Prostate, Urethra, Urine)

The specific qualities of the urine are found in the Urine section. Many of the most useful subrubrics here are found under the rubric "Urination" in the Bladder section. These include "Urination, Involuntary" [enuresis] (659), "Urination, Involuntary, Night" (659), "Urination, Dysuria" [painful urination] (656), "Urination, Dribbling" (655) and "Urination, Frequent" (657). Urinary tract infection symptoms are found in several places but mostly under "Bladder, Inflammation" (646), "Bladder, Urination, Dysuria" (656) and "Urethra, Pain" (673).

Important Rubrics (Bladder Section):

Calculi [stones] (643)
Fullness (645)
Inflammation (646)
Pain (646)
Paralysis (650)
Retention of Urine (650)
Spasm (651)
Tenesmus [urgent need to urinate without being able to do so] (651)
Urging to Urinate (652)
Urination (655)
Weakness (662)

Important Rubrics (Kidney Section):

Heaviness (662)
Inflammation (662)
Pain (663)
Suppression of Urine (666)

Important Rubrics (Prostate Section):

Emission Prostatic Fluid (667)
Enlargement (667)
Induration [hardening] (667)
Inflammation (668)
Pain (668)

Important Rubrics (Urethra Section):

Chordee [painful erection of the penis with curvature] (669)
Constriction (669)
Discharge (669)
Haemorrhage (671)
Inflammation (672)
Itching (672)
Pain (672)
Stricture (679)
Swelling (679)

Important Rubrics (Urine Section):

Bloody (681)
Burning (681)
Cloudy (682)
Color (683)

Copious (685)
Odor (687)
Scanty (688)
Sediment (688)
Sugar (691)

Confusing Terms:

"Addison's Disease" (662) is a chronic adrenal insufficiency characterized by anemia, weakness, low blood pressure, low blood sugar and pigmentation.

"After Lithotomy" (646) refers to after the removal of a kidney stone.

"Casts, Containing" (682) refers to solidification of a liquid poured into a particular mold e.g. the kidney, and therefore showing the structure of the area in which it solidified.

"Catarrh" (643) refers to mucus formation.

"Flocculent" (689) refers to resembling tufts or cottonlike substances and therefore in the urine refers to containing fluffy particles of gray-white mucus.

"Fossa Navicularis" (673) is the terminal dilated portion of the urethra in the penis.

"Indican, Containing" (686) refers to containing potassium salts, which indicates protein breakdown from the intestine.

"Limpid" (686) is clear.

"Neck of Bladder" (646) is the portion of the bladder emptying into the ureters.

"Renal Calculi" (690) are renal stones.

Genitalia, Male

Impotence is found here under "Erections, Incomplete" (695), "Flaccidity" (698) or "Erections, Wanting" (696). Painful erections can be found under "Erections, Painful" (695) but also under "Urethra, Chordee." Both high and low sex drives in men can be found under "Sexual Passion" (711).

Important rubrics:

Coition, Aversion To (693)
Coldness (693)
Condylomata [warts] (693)
Crab-lice (694)
Enlarged (694)
Erections (694)
Eruptions (696)

Excoriation (698)
Flaccidity (698)
Hydrocele [collection of clear fluid in the scrotum] (699)
Induration [hardening of tissue] (699)
Inflammation (699)
Itching (700)
Masturbation Disposition (701)
Numbness (701)
Pain (701)
Redness (709)
Retraction of Penis (709)
Seminal Discharge (709)
Sexual Passion (711)
Swelling (712)
Ulcers (713)
Varicocele (714)

Confusing Terms:

"Blennorrhoea of Glans" (693) refers to a strong mucus discharge, often associated with gonorrhea.

"Constringing" (694) refers to shrinking.

"Elephantiasis Scrotum" (694) is an extreme enlargement and hardening of the scrotum resulting from lymphatic blockage related to worms.

"Empyocele" (694) is a hydrocele that has pus.

"Epididymis" (702) is the duct that connects the testes to the vas deferens.

"Fraenum" (694) is the fold of tissue that limits the movement of the penis.

"Glans" (694) is the tip of the penis.

"Hematocele" (698) is a testicular swelling due to leaking of blood into the testicular sac.

"Onanism" (710) refers to premature withdrawal during intercourse.

"Paraphimosis" (708) is a constricting of the foreskin, preventing it from being drawn forward.

"Perineum" (701) means the area between the scrotum and anus.

"Phimosis" (708) is a narrowing of the opening of the foreskin, preventing it from being drawn backwards.

"Prepuce" (694) is the foreskin.

"Sarcocele" (709) is a tumor of the testes.

"Smegma" (712) is a whitish secretion that collects under the foreskin.

Genitalia, Female

Unfortunately, female genitalia is a tremendously underrepresented section in Kent's *Repertory*. More modern repertories do this section more justice. Symptoms and problems of pregnancy and menses are found here. Yeast infections can be found under "Leucorrhea" (720) and "Itching" (720). Sexual passion can be found here under "Coition" (715), "Desire, Diminished" and "Increased" (717) as well as in the Mind section (see Lesson five). Infertility can also be found here, under "Sterility" (744). Interestingly, there is no corresponding rubric in the Male section. There is a section here for "Menopause" (724). Uterine pain can also be found in the Abdomen section. Ovarian cysts are found under "Tumors, Ovaries, Cysts" (745).

Important Rubrics:

Abortion [refers to spontaneous abortions] (714)
Cancer (715)
Coition [intercourse] (715)
Condylomata [warts] (715)
Contractions [useful for labor] (716)
Displacement of the Uterus (717)
Eruptions (717)
Heat (718)
Heaviness (718)
Inflammation (718)
Itching (720)
Leucorrhea [discharge] (720)
Lochia [discharge of material following childbirth] (723)
Masturbation Disposition (724)
Menopause (724)
Menses (724)
Metrorrhagia [abnormal irregular uterine bleeding] (729)
Numbness (731)
Pain (731)
Placenta Retained (743)
Polypus [benign growths protruding from the uterine wall] (743)
Prolapsed Uterus (743)
Relaxation (744)
Sensitive (744)
Sterility (744)
Swollen (744)
Tumors (745)
Vaginismus (745)

Confusing Terms:

"After Confinement" (743) means after childbirth.

"Atony of Uterus" (715) refers to complete relaxation of the uterus.

"Climaxis" (727) or "Climacteric" (730) refers to menopause.

"Granulation Vagina" (718) is a granular surface often present during healing.

"Nymphomania" (726) means accompanied by an extremely high sex drive.

"Parturition" (737) refers to pregnancy.

"Sacrum" (734) is the tailbone.

"Subinvolution" (744) refers to the uterus remaining excessively large after childbirth.

Larynx and Trachea

Functional qualities of speech, such as stammering, are found under the Mouth section. The most important rubric in this section is "Voice" (758). Here you will find "Hoarseness" (758), "Hoarseness, During Coryza" (750) and "Voice, Lost" (760).

Important Rubrics:

Catarrh [mucous discharge] (746)

Cold (746)

Constriction (746)

Croup [viral infection in children characterized by difficult and noisy respiration and a hoarse cough] (747)

Dryness (748)

Foreign Substance Sensation (748)

Inflammation (748)

Irritation in Air Passages (749)

Laryngismus [spasmodic closure of the throat] (750)

Mucus in the Air Passages (750)

Pain (751)

Paralysis (755)

Roughness (755)

Sensitive Larynx (756)

Swollen (756)

Tickling (757)

Voice (758)

Confusing Terms:

> Epiglottis (748) is a cartilage covered with a mucous membrane at the root of the tongue, which folds back over the opening of the larynx.

Respiration

The most important rubrics in this section are "Asthmatic" (763) and "Difficult" (766). Snoring is here (775). Sleep Apnea Syndrome can be found under "Respiration, Impeded, Night" (763).

Important Rubrics:

> Accelerated (762)
> Anxious (762)
> Arrested (763)
> Asphyxia (763)
> Asthmatic (763)
> Deep (766)
> Difficult (766)
> Impeded or Obstructed (773)
> Irregular (773)
> Loud (774)
> Moaning (774)
> Painful (774)
> Rattling (774)
> Sighing [see also the Mind section] (775)
> Slow (775)
> Snoring (775)
> Wheezing (776)

Confusing Terms:

> "Hay Asthma" (765) is allergic asthma.
> "Stertorous" (776) refers to a loud inspiration occurring in coma or deep sleep.
> "Stridulous" (776) means shrill or harsh.

Notes for Lesson Eight

Quiz for Lesson Eight

Choose the best rubric and page number for the following:

1. My eight-year-old son wets the bed every night.

2. I absolutely hate eggs. I cannot eat them.

3. Because of my recent cold, I have been unable to speak. Nothing comes out.

4. I am always getting yeast infections. I get them after every period.

5. The patient had warts on his scrotum.

6. I have had recurring problems with kidney stones.

7. My daughter's period still hasn't started, even though she is fifteen years old.

8. Ever since I became pregnant, I have been very constipated.

9. The patient has a goiter on the right side.

10. On examining Tom's throat, you find that it has a dark red color.

11. I am the thirstiest person I know. I feel like I can never drink enough.

12. Drinking beer makes me feel nauseous.

13. I feel like I have appendicitis.

14. My teeth hurt every fall.

15. My seventy-five-year-old father has trouble getting his urine started because of his enlarged prostate.

16. My intestines are always making a lot of noise. When I get going, my wife tells me that I sound like a truck.

17. I have bad hemorrhoids that you can't see from the outside.

18. Lately, there has been much undigested food in my stool.

19. My infant son loves to eat sand.

20. My daughter's teeth are very late in developing.

Cough Through Skin

Cough

Important Rubrics:

Time Aggravations (778-781)

Air Aggravates ["Cold" and "Open," amongst others] (780)

Asthmatic (782)

Barking (782)

Chill During (783)

Choking (783)

Cold Aggravates ["Becoming Cold" and "Cold Drinks"] (784)

Constant (784)

Constriction of the Larynx (784)

Croupy [hoarse cough related to a viral infection in children, characterized by difficult and noisy respiration] (785)

Deep (785)

Distressing (786)

Drinking Aggravates (786)

Dry (786)

From Eating (790)

Exhausting (790)

Foreign Body Sensation (791)

Hacking (791)

Hard (793)

Hollow (793)

Inspiration Aggravates (794)

Irritation in Air Passages (794)

Loose (795)

Lying Aggravates (796)

Motion Aggravates (798)

Mucous in Chest (798)

Nervous (798)

Paroxysmal (799)

Persistent (800)

Racking (801)

Rattling (801)

Rising Aggravates (802)

Short (803)

Sleep Aggravates (804)

Spasmodic (804)

Suffocative (806)

Sympathetic (807)

Talking Aggravates (807)

Tickling (807)

Tormenting (809)

Violent (809)

Waking Aggravates (810)

Warm Aggravates(810)

Whooping (810)

Wind Aggravates (811)

Confusing Terms:

"Dyspnea" (788) refers to shortness of breath.

"Fauces" (789) is the throat area.

Expectoration

Important Rubrics:

Time Aggravations (812)

Air Aggravates (812)

Bloody (813)

Copious (814)

Difficult (815)

Easy (815)

Hawked up Mucus (816)

Purulent [Pus-like] (817)

Scanty (818)

Taste (818)

Thick (819)

Tough (820)

Viscid (820)

Confusing Terms:

"Oleaginous" (817) refers to greasy.

"Herbaceous" (819) means green and plantlike in color and texture.

Chest

This section covers the armpit, breastbone, breasts, chest muscles, diaphragm, heart, lungs, ribs, shoulder blade, and sides of the chest. Bronchitis can be found here under "Inflammation, Bronchial Tubes" (835), pleurisy under "Inflammation, Pleura" (836), and pneumonia under "Inflammation, Lungs" (835). Problems pertaining to breast milk can be found under "Milk" (837). Tuberculosis is found under "Phthisis" (878). The Pain section is quite extensive. Breast infections or mastitis can be found under "Chest, Inflammation, Mammae."

Important Rubrics:

Abscess [circumscribed collection of pus] (822)

Angina (822)

Anxiety In (822)

Catarrh [mucousy discharge] (824)

Clothing Aggravates (824)

Coldness (824)

Congestion (825)

Constriction (826)

Cramp (828)

Discoloration (829)

Dropsy [accumulation of fluid often related to heart failure] (829)

Emphysema [chronic lung disease associated with enlargement of the chest and destruction of lung tissue, resulting in shortness of breath] (829)

Eruptions (830)

Excoriation (831)

Fluttering (832)

Fullness (832)

Haemorrhage [bleeding] (833)

Heat Aggravates (834)

Induration [hardening] (835)

Inflammation (835)

Itching (836)

Milk (837)

Murmurs (838)

Oedema Pulmonary [accumulation of fluid in the lungs] (838)

Oppression (838)

Pain (841)

Palpitation (873)

Perspiration (878)

Swelling (880)

Phthisis [tuberculosis] (878)

Sensitive (880)
Spasms (880)
Trembling (881)
Weakness (882)

Confusing Terms:

"Adhesion" (822) refers to parts that stick together after surgery due to inflammation.

"Apex" (848) is the top part of the lung.

"Aphonia" (874) is without voice.

"Atelectasis" (824) means a collapse of a portion of the lung.

"Axilla" (825) is the armpit.

"Costal Cartilages" (853) are cartilage that connect the ribs to the sternum.

"Diaphragm" (835) is the muscle that separates the abdomen from the chest.

"Empyema" (830) is the accumulation of pus around the lungs.

"Exudation in Valves of Heart" (832) refers to oozing of fluid from the valves. This is also known as endocarditis.

"Endocardium" (835) is the membrane covering the inside of the heart.

"Hepatization of the Lungs" (834) refers to the change during pneumonia of lung tissue into a firm jellylike substance the consistency of liver.

"Hydrothorax" (827) is the accumulation of water in the lungs.

"Lactiferous Tubes" (846) are milk ducts.

"Mammae" (822) are the breasts.

"Pectoral Muscles" (845) are chest muscles.

"Percussion Aggravates" (861) refers to tapping on the chest during a physical exam.

"Pericardium" (835) is the membrane that surrounds the heart.

"Praecordial Region" (870) refers to the heart.

"Scapula" (845) is the shoulder blade.

"Stenocardia" (880) refers to angina.

"Sternum" (825) is the breast bone.

Back

The back is divided into five separate sections: cervical (neck), dorsal/thoracic (midback), lumbar (lower back), sacral (tailbone), and coccyx (tailbone). The Pain rubric is the largest in this section. Sciatica can be found in a variety of places, but mostly in the Extremities section under "Pain, Lower Limbs, Sciatica" (1064) and "Extremities, Pain, Crural Nerves" (1071).

Important Rubrics:

Coldness (884)
Concussion of Spine (886)
Cracking (887)
Curvature of Spine [scoliosis] (887)
Eruptions (887)
Heat (890)
Heaviness (891)
Inflammation (892)
Injuries of Spine (892)
Itching (892)
Numbness (893)
Opisthotonos [arching of head backwards and spine forwards as if the
    head were to touch the toes] (893)
Pain (894)
Perspiration (944)
Spasms (946)
Stiffness (946)
Straining Easily (947)
Tension (948)
Weakness (950)

Confusing Terms:

Bifida (884) is a birth defect related to defects in the bony structure sur-
    rounding the spine, causing the protrusion of the spinal cord onto the
    surface.
Emprosthotonos (887) refers to muscle spasms in which the head and
    spine are flexed forward.
Glutei Muscles (908) are the muscles of the buttocks.
Nates (909) refers to the buttocks.
Psoas (884) is a muscle that goes from the thigh into the lumbar spine.
Pubis (909) is the anterior most part of the hip bones.
Sacro Iliac Symphysies (934) is the area where the tailbone and the hip
    connect.

Extremities

The Extremities section is the largest section of the *Repertory*. The general layout of the section begins with the upper limbs, working down the arms to the fingers, and then moves to the lower limbs, working down the legs to the toes. There are also separate listings here for "Muscles," "Joints," "Nails," and "Tendons." The first finger is the index finger. Flexor muscles are those that flex or bend the part. Extensor muscles similarly extend the part. Abduction is movement away from the midline of the body. Adduction is movement towards the midline. Supination is turning over so that the arm or palm faces upwards. Pronation is the opposite. Clumsiness is found here under "Awkwardness" (953). Sciatica can be found under "Pain, Lower Limbs, Sciatica" (1064) and "Extremities, Pain, Curual Nerves" (1071).

Important Rubrics:

    Abscess [localized collection of pus in a cavity] (952)
    Arthritic Nodosities [hard lumps deep under the skin; related to arthritis] (952)
    Awkwardness [clumsiness] (953)
    Brittle Nails (954)
    Bunions (954)
    Chilliness (955)
    Chorea [writhing, dancelike movements] (956)
    Clenching (956)
    Coldness (956)
    Constriction (965)
    Contraction (966)
    Convulsions (968)
    Corns (969)
    Cracks of Skin (970)
    Cracking in Joints (970)
    Cramps (971)
    Discoloration (978)
    Dislocation (983)
    Dryness (984)
    Eruption (986)
    Felon [infection around the nail bed] (1005)
    Formification (1006)
    Hanging Down (1009)
    Heat (1010)
    Heaviness (1013)
    Hip Joint Disease (1017)
    Incoordination (1017)
    Inflammation (1018)
    Injuries (1019)
    Inversion (1019)
    Jerkiness (1029)
    Motion (1033)
    Numbness (1035)
    Pain (1043)

Paralysis (1176)
Perspiration (1181)
Restlessness (1187)
Sensitive (1189)
Stiffness (1191)
Swelling (1196)
Tension (1202)
Trembling (1210)
Twitching (1215)
Ulcers (1220)
Varices [enlarged torturous veins] (1223)
Warts (1223)
Weakness (1224)

Confusing Terms:

"Anchylosis" (952) is an immobility and unusual stiffness.

"Ankle Malleolus" (962) is the bony prominence on the sides of the elbow joint.

"Ataxia" (953) is a lack of muscular coordination manifesting in abnormal gait.

"Biceps," "Deltoids," and "Triceps" (1055) are the three muscles of the arm.

"Bursae" (954) is a saclike cavity between joints.

"Callosities" (954) are incomplete healings of fractures where new growth is occurring.

"Chilblains" (955) are rednesses of the extremities associated with burning and itching when it becomes cold.

"Endocarditis" (1198) is an inflammation of the inside of the heart or its valves.

"External Condyle of Elbow" (1084) is the tip of the elbow.

"Femur" (954) is the long bone of the thigh.

"Fibula" (955) is the calf bone.

"Ganglion on Wrist" (1009) is a cyst containing fibrous tissue on the wrist.

"Hemiplegia" (1176) is a paralysis of only one side of the body.

"Humerus" (954) is the main bone of the upper arm.

"Inversion of Foot" (1019) means turning inward.

"Metacarpal" (1024) refers to the middle bone of the fingers.

"Milk Leg" (1033) refers to inflammation of veins of the leg post partum.

"Nates" (954) are the buttocks.

"Os Calcis" (1007) refers to the heel bone.

"Patella" (954) is the knee cap.

"Popliteus" (954) is the posterior part of the knee.

"Olecranon" (958) is the tip of the elbow.

"Periosteum" (1018) is the membrane surrounding a bone.

"Phalanx" (1061) is a finger or toe.

"Popliteus" (1183) is the back of the knee.

"Radius" and "Ulna" (1057) are the bones of the forearm.

"Shoulder Acromion" (1010) is the highest part of the shoulder blade.

"Synovitis" (1018) refers to an inflammation of the sac that surrounds the joints.

"Tendo Achillis" (976) is the achilles tendon.

"Tibia" (954) is the shin bone.

"Ulnar Nerve" (1157) is the nerve that controls the inside of the arm.

"Ulnar Side of Hand"(973) is the inside of the hand with the little finger.

"Wrist Radial Side" (993) is the outside of the hand along the thumb.

Sleep

"Dreams" (1235) are found here. In some modern repertories, the Dream rubric is found in the Mind section. "Somnambulism" (81) and "Talking in Sleep" (86) are found in the Mind section. "Nightmares" (1242) are found here. "Sleeplessness" (1251) is another important rubric here. "Yawning" (1256) is also found in this section.

Important Rubrics:

Deep (1234)

Disturbed (1235)

Heavy (1246)

Position [various positions of sleep] (1246)

Restless (1247)

Sleepiness (1248)

Sleeplessness (1251)

Unrefreshing (1255),

Waking (1255)

Yawning (1256)

Chill

Important Rubrics:

Coldness (1259)

Time Modalities (1259)

Open Air (1262)

Beginning in and Extending from [various parts of the body] (1263)

Chilliness (1264)

Creeping (1266)
Drinking (1266)
Eating (1267)
External (1267)
Internal (1268)
Shaking (1270)
Sides (1272)
Single Parts (1272)
Times (1272)

Confusing Terms:

"Autumn Chill" (1262) refers to every seven days.
"Quartan" (1270) refers to every fourth day.
"Quotidian" (1270) is a daily chill.
"Tertian" (1262) refers to every third day.

Fever

Important Rubrics:

Heat (1278)
Time Modalities (1278)
Alternating with Chills (1280)
Bed, in (1281)
Burning Heat (1283)
Cerebrospinal [useful for meningitis] (1282)
Continued (1284)
Exanthematic Fevers [fever associated with a skin eruption] (1286)
External (1286)
Intense (1287)
Intermittent [periods of normal temperature] (1288)
Internal (1288)
Puerperal [during childbirth] (1289)
Relapsing [gets well but then relapses] (1289)
Remittent [periods of improvement without recovery] (1289)
Septic [infection of the blood] (1290)
Side (1290)
Succession of Stages (1291)
Uncovering (1292)

Confusing Terms:

"Autumnal" (1281) refers to every seven days.
"Gastric Fever" (1287) means associated with gastritis.

"Hectic" (1287) refers to constant.

"Hemorrhagic" (1285) or Manchurian Fever has an unknown cause and is associated with fever, headache, chills, abdominal pain, nausea, and vomiting and ultimately bleeding.

"Yellow Fever" (1292) is an infectious disease caused by a mosquito that is associated with high fever, bloody vomiting, and jaundice.

"Zymotic Fevers" (1292) are fevers that are associated with infectious disease.

Perspiration

Important Rubrics:

Perspiration (1293)

Time Modalities [especially at night] (1293)

Anxiety During (1295)

Clammy (1295)

Cold (1296)

Hot (1297)

Odor (1298)

Profuse (1299)

Sides (1300)

Single Parts (1301)

Sleep (1301)

Symptoms Aggravate (1302)

Skin

Scarlet fever is found here under "Eruptions, Scarlet" (1318) as well as under "Fever, Exanthematic, Scarlatina" (1286). Similarly, measles is found under "Skin, Eruptions, Measles" (1314) as well as "Fever, Exanthematic, Measles" (1286). Poison ivy and poison oak can be found under "Eruptions, Rhus Poisoning" (1318). Jaundice is found under "Discoloration, Yellow" (1307).

Important Rubrics:

Anaesthesia (1303)

Burning (1303)

Chapping (1304)

Cracks (1305)

Discoloration (1305)

Dry (1307)

Ecchymoses [bruising] (1308)

Eruptions (1308)

Erysipelas [superficial contagious skin infection with fever, shiny red swollen lesions caused by Beta Hemolytic Streptococcus] (1324)
Formication [creepy crawly sensation, like insects on skin] (1325)
Heat without fever (1326)
Inflammation (1326)
Itching (1327)
Moles (1330)
Numbness (1330)
Sensitiveness (1331)
Sore, Becomes [decubitus ulcer] (1331)
Stings of Insects (1331)
Swelling (1331)
Ulcers (1333)
Warts (1339)

Confusing Terms:

"Carbuncle" (1310) is a large and deep abscess in which there is a circumscribed collection of pus.
"Cicatrices" (1304) refers to fibrous scar tissue replacing normal healthy tissue. This is an other name for keloids.
"Condylomata" (1324) are warts.
"Ecthyma" (1312) is a skin disease that is associated with large pustules that ulcerate and crust over.
"Erysipelatous" (1320) is an inflammation of the skin associated with fever.
"Hidebound Sensation" (1326) refers to tension of the skin.
"Ichthyosis" (1319) refers to dry scaly skin, like fish scales.
"Intertrigo" (1327) is chafing of the skin.
"Lenticular" (1307) refers to skin that has a crystalline appearance.
"Lupus" (1330) refers to tuberculosis of the skin.
"Nodules" (1304) are hard lumps deep under the skin.
"Petechiae" (1315) are small pinpoints of bleeding in the skin.
"Pemphigus" (1315) is a severe skin disease with blister formation that develop in crops.
"Pocks" (1316) are pustular eruptions of the skin.
"Psoriasis Diffusa" (1316) is a form of psoriasis where the lesions are confluent.
"Roseola" (1318) is any rose colored eruption.
"Rupia" (1318) refers to ulcers of late syphilis covered with yellow brown crusts similar in shape to oyster shells.
"Sarcomatous Ulcers" (1337) are cancerous ulcers.

"Sudamina" (1323) are minute blisters caused by the retention of fluid in a sweat follicle.

"Tubercles" (1320) are round nodules associated with tuberculosis.

"Varicose Ulcers" (1339) are ulcers associated with swollen veins.

"Vesicles" (1304) are small, watery blisters.

"Wens" (1340) are sebaceous cysts.

Notes for Lesson Nine

Quiz for Lesson Nine

Choose the best rubric and page number for the following:

1. I get this severe pounding in my chest whenever I get upset.
2. Whenever my son gets really angry, his head arches backwards and his spine arches forwards like a spasm.
3. I have a bad cough that comes on every time I breathe in.
4. I have recurring dreams of events that happened in my childhood.
5. My wife is very clumsy with her hands.
6. I get chilled easily in the back of my neck.
7. My feet get colder than "the North Pole in January."
8. My daughter has nightmares every night.
9. I have problems with severe night sweats.
10. I have ugly white spots on my nails.
11. My husband cannot keep his legs still while he is sleeping.
12. I just got stung by a wasp.
13. I have a creepy, crawly, itchy feeling in my armpit.
14. My skin gets very red with streaks after I scratch it.
15. I get a chill every third day.
16. I cannot sleep on my left side.
17. I cannot stop yawning after I eat.
18. I have an itchy rash that my doctor says is shingles.
19. Whenever I hear someone else coughing, I have to cough.
20. I get cramps in my calves every night.

Case Analysis

General Comments

There are as many ways to analyze a case as there are homeopaths to analyze them. The methods range from a complex computerized analysis to dowsing, from a deep, essence-level understanding of the person to prescribing based on pathology. Ultimately, the best method is one that leads you to a good result. The best homeopaths are flexible. Rather than limiting themselves to a single method, they adapt their methods to the case at hand. The goal is to produce consistently reliable results in prescribing.

It is necessary to match the complexity of the patient's being with the complexity of the remedy. In actual fact, case analysis is a bit of a misnomer. Case synthesis might be a better term. The process is often about taking a great deal of disparate information and bringing it together into a meaningful whole.

The struggle that many beginning homeopaths have with case analysis is with the perception of what is most characteristic in a case vs. what is common. Common symptoms seldom help you find the remedy. The symptom of pain in the ear is common to ear infections and is not particularly useful in finding the right remedy. However, the symptom of pain in the ear that is much better with boring the finger into the ear is more peculiar and speaks to the person rather than the disease. This requires a basic knowledge of common symptoms of specific diseases, which comes through clinical experience.

When the solution to a case eventually presents itself, there is an internal feeling that is present in the homeopath. Things click together suddenly and there is a satisfied feeling, like an "ah ha." Various people experience this differently. It is the moment when everything suddenly comes into focus.

Analyzing a case can sometimes be a daunting task. It is helpful to remember that you are never alone in this process. The work of all the other homeopaths precedes you. If there is a willingness on your part, they will be with you in your endeavor.

In analyzing a case, it is often helpful to look for essence, totality, and characteristic symptoms. Essence is more three-dimensional, totality two-dimensional and characteristic symptoms are one-dimensional. The best possible scenario is when all three elements are present in a case that all fit a particular remedy. When this occurs, you can prescribe the remedy with confidence. Often when all three are present, it is a sign of a strong vitality, or having a strong vital force.

Wonder

The capacity to fully analyze a case involves the ability to wonder. The most common mistake of beginning homeopathic prescribers in case analysis is to come up with an idea of what to prescribe early in a case and then to proceed to prove that their idea is correct. With the right questioning, you can prove that almost any remedy is a correct prescription. It is easy to get stuck on a particular remedy and not allow yourself to see the myriad of other possibilities in a case. Wondering is about the ability to exercise our imaginations as freely and fully as possible, considering all possible approaches to a case. It is important to allow your imagination to roam freely, with the proviso that the imagination is always anchored in what the patient says.

When you think of a particular remedy during casetaking, it is best to write it down and then let it go and move on. A useful exercise to use when you become convinced of a particular remedy is to ask yourself what you would give if the particular remedy you have in mind was given and did not work. Another approach is to look intently for a better remedy than the one you have in mind. When you start focusing on a particular remedy in your mind, you take your attention off the patient and stop listening as deeply. For beginning homeopaths, it is best not to think about any remedies during the case and to only begin to analyze the case afterwards.

Wonder is also an attitude that we hold within ourselves. When we come to our work with an attitude of wonder and awe, we open ourselves to the myriad of possibilities that life has to offer. It is a childlike place.

Essence

Essence is difficult to define. There is no single way to describe it, and words are often inadequate. It is something that is caught and perceived on a different level. It refers to a deeper level that contains a whole truth to something (gestalt). It involves seeing the whole rather than the parts. It is the single golden thread, or the music that runs through a case. It is the center of the case from which all else springs. Rajan Sankaran describes this as the "core delusion" (fixed false belief), from which all the symptoms arise. Edward Whitmont describes this as a form pattern which arises out of the dynamic field of the individual. Perception of the essence of something is similar to looking into a two-dimensional picture of wavy lines (popularized in contemporary art) and all of a sudden having a three dimensional image appear. The picture becomes alive in a new and exciting way, and there is a feeling of suddenly grasping the whole.

Essence prescribing has become increasingly prevalent in the last twenty-five years. In the past, many of the prescriptions were made based on a physical understanding of the case, accompanied by its general characteristics. As the health of our planet has deteriorated and suppression of the vital force has increased through pollution and allopathic drugging, the center of gravity of cases has been pushed deeper in the individual and more into the emotional and mental plane. Accordingly, the emotional and mental symptoms have become increasingly important in prescribing over time. It is not always possible to perceive the essence in a case, but when it is present this can be quite helpful in prescribing. Not all of the essences of the various remedies are known or understood.

For example, George Vithoulkas describes the essence of the remedy *Alumina* as having partly to do with constipation. On the physical level this has to do with obdurate, severe constipation with great dryness of the rectum. On the emotional level this has to do with apathy, listlessness, indifference, and laziness. On the mental level this encompasses slowing of the mental faculties, dullness, confusion, hazy thinking, and slowness in responses to questioning.

Another example is the essence of *Rhus toxicodendron,* which has to do with motion/stiffness. On the physical level there is extreme restlessness, restless sleep at night, better from initial motion and worse from overexertion. On the emotional level there is irritability, joking, desire to be carried fast (children), hurriedness, and impatience. On the mental level there is restlessness, jumping from one topic to another, inability to sleep because of restless thoughts, and a dullness of the mind that improves on motion. It is also an important remedy for attention deficit disorder.

The following is a case that is illustrative of the idea of essence (for a discussion of underlining, e.g., (2), see Lesson Four). M.W. is a thirty-two-year-old male complaining of an acute cold over the last five days, which is gradually getting worse. There were no specific precipitants. There is frequent sneezing (2) and recurrent bouts of sneezing (2). He says that he is sneezing so much that he is "afraid my nose will fall off." There is itching of the nose (2). He has a dry cough (1) that is worse in the morning. He has an acrid and thin nasal discharge (2), which he is fearful "is disfiguring my nose," although there is no evidence of this on observation. He has a sore throat that improves with warm drinks (2). He desires sweets (1) and lemon (2). There are swollen glands of the neck (2). He complains of left knee pain (1). There is a fear of throat cancer since the onset of the cold (2). He cannot be talked out of this fear and wants to see an ear/nose/throat specialist, although there are no specific symptoms that would precipitate such a referral. He is chilly (2) and has a hoarse voice (1–2). There is a sweetish taste in the mouth (1–2) and perspiration on the face.

The central theme/essence of this case has to do with erroneous ideas about his body and his body's health. The remedy that most closely matches this essence is the remedy Sabadilla. This can be found under the rubric "Mind, Delusions, Body, Erroneous Ideas As to the State of His" (p. 22). He was given Sabadilla 30C in two doses four hours apart and all of his symptoms resolved within twelve hours. Later he said, "I was in an altered state. I have no idea why I had this idea about throat cancer. It doesn't make any sense now, but it seemed so strong at the time." There was no recurrence of any of these symptoms.

Totality

Once a case has been taken, the next step is to evaluate the totality of the patient's symptoms. Often this takes the form of outlining the most important symptoms in the case. The ones that are given the most importance are the ones that are the most peculiar and intense and reflect the whole person. Symptoms that most limit the individual's freedom should be included.

The totality of symptoms is more of a two-dimensional way of prescribing. It involves identifying the sum totality of all of the symptoms of a case and then finding the remedy that most closely matches that totality. This is a method that lends itself best to repertorization. Symptoms that are included in the totality are ones that are most true of the person and not necessarily of the disease or the pathology. Mental and general symptoms often figure more prominently in the analysis than physical symptoms.

An example is the following case. D.F. is a sixteen-year-old male who has had the flu for the last week, with nausea and vomiting and intermittent mild stomach pain. He had mostly recovered yesterday, but today his parents call saying that he has developed severe abdominal pain (3) in the last two hours, which started at nine p.m. They are thinking of sending him to the emergency room, as they are worried about appendicitis, but are willing to give you one try to find the right remedy. The pain is stitching in character (2) and predominantly on the right side of the abdomen (2). He is very thirsty for cold drinks (3), but vomits immediately after drinking. The pain is worse with motion (2). He has been having diarrhea every morning when he gets up (2). He is quite irritable (2–3). There is no fever.

	Bry.	Bell.	Calc.	Caust.	Cham	Nux-v	Ars.	Ip.
TOTAL	14	10	9	9	9	8	8	8
RUBRICS	5	4	4	4	4	5	4	4
1. Abdomen; PAIN; stitching	3	2	2	2	2	2	2	3
2. Mind; IRRITABILITY	3	3	3	3	3	3	2	2
3. Stomach; DESIRES; cold drink	3	2	2	2	3	1	3	
4. VOMITING; General; drinking; cold water, after	2					1	1	1
5. Stomach; PAIN; General; motion, on	3	3	2	2	1	1		2

The repertorization analysis lies above. Based on the totality of symptoms, *Bryonia alba* was chosen. He was given 30C every fifteen minutes for two hours and the symptoms completely resolved. There was a mild recurrence of symptoms on the following evening, which quickly responded to the repeating of the remedy in a single dosage, and there was no further recurrence of symptoms. This case illustrates the totality approach to case analysis.

Characteristic Symptoms

Characteristic symptoms are ones that call to mind a particular remedy. These may take a variety of forms, including keynotes; pace of onset symptoms; "as if" symptoms; strange, rare, and peculiar symptoms; alternating symptoms; periodical symptoms, and concomitants. Prescribing based solely on these characteristic symptoms is a more one-dimensional type of prescribing. The most helpful characteristic symptoms are ones that reveal the core of the person.

A *keynote* symptom is defined as a characteristic fact or idea about a remedy. For example, putting the feet out of the covers at night because they are too hot is a keynote of the remedy *Sulphur*. A craving for soft-boiled eggs is a keynote of the remedy *Calcarea carbonica*. This should be distinguished from a confirmatory symptom, which substantiates a remedy choice but is less strongly characteristic of a particular remedy. For example, a craving for sweets is a keynote of the remedy *Lycopodium* and a confirmatory symptom of the remedy *Calcarea carbonica*, although there are many other remedies that have this symptom. A number of authors have published books in which keynote and confirmatory symptoms are listed, such as Morrison's *Desktop Guide to Keynotes and Confirmatory Symptoms* and Allen's *Keynotes of the Materia Medica*.

Another form that characteristic symptoms take are *"as if"* symptoms. These tend to be strong and very descriptive symptoms of a particular remedy. An example would be a young man who has such major migraine headaches that it feels "as if" the top of his head would blow off. Another example is the symptom "as if" there was the rustling of a grasshopper in the left ear. There are several books available on these symptoms as well, the most well known being Roberts' *Sensations As If*.

Strange, rare and peculiar symptoms are ones that are not characteristic of the particular disease but are characteristic of the particular patient. They often are paradoxical symptoms, i.e., are contradictory in nature. An example is a strong fever accompanied by thirstlessness, or a great coldness of the foot that is much better from cold bathing. Often these symptoms can be found in the repertory as the only remedy listed for a particular rubric.

Pace of onset is another form of characteristic symptom. Some remedy states come on quite slowly, as in *Bryonia alba* and *Gelsemium sempivirens*, whereas others come on with great suddenness, intensity, and violence, like *Aconite napellus*, *Belladonna*, and *Cantharis*.

Alternating symptoms are ones that alternate from one organ system to another, for example, diarrhea alternating with arthritis or skin eruptions alternating with fever. Some remedy states show a certain periodicity.

Periodicity refers to occurring at regular intervals. For example, the remedy *Cedron* is well known for its ability to produce complaints at the exact same time every day (p. 1391).

Concomitants are symptoms that occur at the same time as the chief complaint. An example of a concomitant would be a migraine headache that is always accompanied by rheumatic pain in the left ankle.

Here is a case that was analyzed based on characteristic symptoms. N.A. is a twenty-eight-year-old female who has sprained her back while heavy lifting seven days ago (2). The pain is dull and aching in character. It is worse from touch (1) and worse from heat (1). The pain is in the central part of the lumbar back. There is no past history of back problems. There is mild redness (1) and swelling (1) in the area. She needs to sleep on her side because of the pain. The pain is worse in the morning on waking but gets better as the day goes on. She is mildly more thirstless than usual. She has a craving for sweets. There is a sensation in the back, as if cold water was poured on the area. She took *Arnica montana* 30C, *Rhus toxicodendron* 30C, and *Ruta graveolens* 30C without any improvement.

This is a case where many of the symptoms are common and not characteristic of the individual. A craving for sweets is common in our culture and should not be used as a symptom unless it is quite strong. What is characteristic about the case is the sensation of cold water being poured on the back (p. 885). Based on this symptom, the remedy *Pulsatilla* 30C was prescribed. There was steady improvement after the remedy and symptoms resolved in twenty-four hours. There was no recurrence of symptoms.

Confirmatory Questions

Once the case has been taken and analyzed, a number of remedy possibilities may become apparent. At this point it can be helpful to ask confirmatory questions. Confirmatory questions are questions that help to confirm or deny particular remedies. These are available in many books (e.g., *Desktop Guide to Keynotes and Confirmatory Symptoms*, by Roger Morrison). Caution should be used, however, that you don't try to confirm the remedy before you have finished fully taking and analyzing the case.

Etiology

Etiology means causation. Etiology is a useful tool in analyzing cases. It is always important to discover how a condition or state originated. At times people are not able to remember the inciting cause, but often the originating story can give you a significant clue into the nature of the remedy. Whenever you hear the story that "I have never been well since…," etiology is an important case analysis technique to consider. Foubister, in his book *Tutorials on Homeopathy,* has an excellent chapter on "The Significance of Past History," which explores this concept further. Examples in the *Repertory* include the following:

Ailments from Admonition (1)
Ailments from Anger (2)
Ailments from Anticipation (4)
Ailments from Bad News (9)
Ailments from Cares and Worries (10)
Ailments after Drinking (37)
Ailments from Egotism (39)
Ailments from Embarrassment (39)
Ailments from Excitement (40)
Ailments from Fright (49)
Ailments from Grief (51)
Ailments from Homesickness (51)
Ailments from Wounded Honor (52)
Ailments from Indignation (55)
Ailments from Joy (60)
Ailments from Being Looked at (63)
Ailments from Disappointed Love (63)
Ailments from Fine Manual Work (64)
Ailments from Moonlight (68)
Ailments from Mortification (68)
Ailments from Reproaches (68)
Ailments from Rudeness of Others (75)
Ailments from Being Scorned (78)
Ailments from Sexual Excesses (79)
Ailments from Pleasant Surprises (85)
Ailments from Mental Work (95)
Suppression of Discharges (1404)
Vaccinosis [problems that develop after a vaccination] (1410)

Here is a case example. G.M. is a six-year-old boy who hasn't been well since a vaccination three weeks ago. Prior to that time he had been in good health. He has had symptoms of a cold since the vaccination. These include cough (1–2), pale green coryza (1–2), swollen, painful lymph nodes (1), sore throat (1–2), and a mild fever of 100 degrees. He is mildly irritable. There have been three warts that have developed on his left hand in the last two weeks.

The cold symptoms here are fairly nondescript. What stands out about this case is the etiology ("Generalities, Vaccinosis" p. 1410). This information, coupled with the warts of the hand ("Extremities, Warts, Hand" p. 1223) led to a prescription of *Thuja occidentalis* 12C. He took this three times within twenty-four hours and the symptoms completely resolved with no recurrence.

Kingdoms/Family

For many years in homeopathy, each remedy was considered and studied separately, with little correlation between one remedy and another. Recently, there has been a growing appreciation that certain families of remedies share characteristics. This is an analysis strategy that has been around for some time (Farrington, et al.) but has only been popularized in recent years through the work of Rajan Sankaran. In Sankaran's *Soul of Remedies,* he has many charts that illustrate these ideas further.

One common characteristic between remedies is that of a family. For example, there are certain qualities that all snake remedies have in common, such as jealousy, passion, loquacity, fear of snakes, fear of water and intolerance of clothes around the neck. There are certain qualities that metals have, such as a focus on performance, need for control and fear/dreams of heights.

Another form that this can take is through the study of salt remedies. If we know something about the element magnesium and something about the element iodine (iodatum), then we can extrapolate to understand something about the remedy *Magnesia iodatum.* The salt will always be more than its constituent parts, but will still have symptoms of the respective parts. Similarly, Jan Scholten has recently written about the periodic table of elements (a grouping of the elements by atomic number and weight). He feels that if we understand a particular element on the periodic table, then elements that lie in proximity to that element on the table or in the same grouping will have similar characteristics (*Homeopathy and the Elements,* by Jan Scholten).

There are four kingdoms of remedies: animals, plants, minerals, and imponderables (for definition of imponderabilia see Appendix M). Animal remedies tend to have energy towards attraction. There is often a split between one side of themselves and the other: one side may be affectionate and warm, caring and playful, while the other is competitive, jealous, and aggressive. Aggression is a common theme, as is the theme of survival. They can be flashy dressers and want to attract attention. Their behavior is often attention-seeking. They tend to be lively, vivacious, and animated. They maintain good eye contact and make strong human contact. There is a desire for company. They are often focused on appearance. There are dreams of animals, pursuit, attack, love, and flying. There may be a fear of being attacked. There are often animal patterns in their dress or in their jewelry.

Plant remedies have a theme of sensitivity to the environment. They need to be able to respond to changes in the environment. They prefer flowery patterns or irregular patterns in their dress. They present their complaints in a disorganized fashion and often don't describe their symptoms completely. Their complaints are rapid in onset and have a changing nature. Their feelings are most important to them, and they may fear being hurt. They are sensitive, soft, emotional people who are easily affected and may have abrupt mood changes. They may have dreams of plants, greenery, nature, music, and art. There often is a great love of plants in their life.

The mineral remedy focus is on structure. They tend to be quite organized. They often wear plain clothes or clothes in symmetrical patterns, stripes, or checks. They will present complaints in chronological order and have only one or two complaints. They may bring extensive notes. They use a lot of figures and numbers in their speech. They tend to have chronic complaints of a slow, progressive nature.

Here is a case example. O.W. is a forty-five-year-old woman who complains of having a sore throat (2–3) for the last ten days. She saw her family physician, who did a strep throat culture, which was negative, and who told her that it was just a virus and that there was nothing that he could do. The symptoms are worse on the left side of the throat (2). Her throat pain is worse when swallowing, eating, drinking, and talking. The pain is described as "burning" (2) and "stitching" (2). There is a slight cough that is associated with the sore throat. She states that she cannot stand to have anything touch her neck (2) and feels a sense of constriction there (2). She notes that she has been much more irritable and sarcastic lately. Her husband states that "she keeps striking at me" and that this is a distinct change from her usual state. She has been jealous of her husband's attention lately (1–2). The symptoms started after she encountered a snake while running ten days ago. The only emotion that she felt at the time was fascination/mesmerization, but she could not remember what type of snake it was. The symptoms started within minutes after the encounter. Since that time she has had recurrent dreams of "jungle snakes" nearly every night.

The throat symptoms here are fairly nondescript. What stands out about the case is the snake energy that is present. The jealousy, constriction at the throat, aggressive striking quality, snake dreams, and the mesmerization are all qualities of snakes. I chose *Lachesis* 30C because of the left-sided symptoms and because it needed to be for a jungle snake (*Lachesis* is from the Amazon). She was given three doses and her symptoms resolved completely in twenty-four hours. There was no recurrence of any symptoms, and her snake dreams resolved.

Doctrine of Signatures

The "Doctrine of Signatures" is an idea that has been present for many centuries but was popularized by Paracelsus. He said "God would not place a disease upon the Earth without providing a cure for it, and a clue to the cure's identity. He places a signature upon it by making remedies resemble the organs or maladies that they can cure." The idea is that there is a correspondence between the substance itself and what it can heal.

Here are some examples of the Doctrine of Signatures as it applies to remedies. The plant thorn-apple grows in disturbed soil and often in graveyards. The remedy *Stramonium* (thorn-apple) is the main remedy for fear of cemeteries. The honey bee tends to be quite active and protective of his hive. The remedy *Apis mellifica* (honey bee) also is quite busy (10) and jealously protective of its family (60). The metal platinum is one of the most valuable metals, set above all others. The remedy *Platinum metallicum* is one of our most haughty (p. 51) of remedies, considering themselves superior to others.

This idea can be utilized in case analysis. A patient may come to you, and no known remedy seems to fit the case. When you analyze the case, you see that the person exhibits certain characteristics that remind you of a particular substance in nature that has never been proven. This may be the correct remedy for the case.

Here is an example. J.T. is a four-year-old boy who has developed colicky abdominal pain (2) over the last few weeks. He was given a variety of remedies without response, including *Chamomilla, Belladonna, Cina,* and *Colocynthis.* He would vomit on occasion (1) but mostly lacked appetite. The pains would cause him to bend double (2). He was also constipated (1–2). With the pains he was extremely restless (2–3) and, according to his parents, would "flit from room to room." He was irritable (2) and without provocation at times would run up to his parents and bite them, drawing blood (3). He was very impatient (2) and would quarrel with anything his parents said (2). The only other thing that the parents noticed was that he would often make a humming/droning kind of noise when he got the colicky pains.

When I restudied the case, what stood out to me was the great restlessness, flitting from room to room, the biting to the point of drawing blood, and the droning noise that he made with the pain. When I put this all together I thought of the mosquito, which is the remedy *Culex musca.* We know very little about this remedy, although it is described as impatient, restless, and quarrelsome on the slightest provocation. Based on the Doctrine of Signatures, I gave him a single dosage of *Culex* 30C. He had an immediate improvement of symptoms following the remedy. There was a mild relapse several days later. The remedy had to be repeated once more, and he did well. There was no further recurrence of symptoms after that. I chose *Culex* over other stinging insects (e.g., *Apis*) because of the drawing of blood.

Pathology

Pathological prescriptions involve using the most common remedy for a particular pathology. This is the most common method for first aid prescribing, e.g., *Thuja occidentalis* is used for warts and *Cantharis* is used for urinatry tract infections.

Thinking in this way, however, is somewhat limited, as for example, *Arnica montana* is used for much more than bruising and *Calendula officinalis* for more than cuts. The risk with this type of prescribing is "suppression," in which a superficial remedy is chosen that is effective, but at the cost of suppressing the symptom deeper into the organism. This especially happens in cases with a weak vital force. There are also a variety of pathologies in which it is very difficult to say which are the most common remedies. Many authors have written books in which the most common remedies are listed for particular conditions (e.g., *Homeopathic Therapeutics* by Lilienthal). Pathological prescribing may also be the only choice in critical situations such as coma, where it is impossible to get much of a case.

Here is an illustrative case of prescribing based on pathology. C.L. is an eight-year-old girl who was brought to me for fatigue (2) and a large wart on the tip of her nose (3). These symptoms had persisted over three to four weeks. I spent over two hours with her and her family and could not elicit *any* other symptoms.

I prescribed a single dose of *Causticum* 30C. *Causticum* is almost a specific remedy for warts on the tip of the nose (354), although the remedy *Aethusa* also has this symptom. The wart fell off in twenty-four hours and her energy significantly improved. There was no evidence of any recurrence of these symptoms.

Miasms

The concept of miasm is a concept originated by Samuel Hahnemann. He developed this idea in an effort to explain chronic disease. In his practice he found that often remedies would work effectively but that frequently these symptoms would recur. The remedies that he was giving did not change the underlying predisposition to disease. Miasms are infectious and passed from generation to generation. They have a capacity to enter into the pattern of vitality of the organism. They cause a specific predisposition to disease.

There are three factors that point to the presence of a miasm in a case. The first is age. Conditions that begin at birth are often miasmatic. The second is family history. When you hear of a multigenerational pattern of specific recurrent problems, you immediately think of a miasm. For example, a strong multigenerational history of early cardiac disease is suggestive of the sycotic miasm. The third factor is individual characteristics of a case that point to a specific miasm. For example, congenital abnormalities such as harelip and clubfoot often point to the syphilitic miasm.

Hahnemann described three main miasms: *psoric, sycotic,* and *syphilitic.* The psoric miasm often involves weakness, fatigue, skin eruptions, and allergies. *Sulphur* and *Psorinum* are good examples of this miasm.

The sycotic miasm has an energy that is overabundant and flows outward. There is extroversion. Frequently there are warts, tumors, growths, and much discharge. They tend to be worse from suppression of the discharge. They feel better in the evening. They are worse from damp weather. There is often a strong family history of heart disease, dysfunctional families, and sexual pathology. *Medorrhinum* and *Thuja occidentalis* are good examples of remedies for this miasm.

The syphilitic miasm has an energy that turns inward and is destructive. Often there are bone pains, introversion, destructive ulceration of tissues, and suicidal depression. The patients tend to be worse at night and better in the daylight. Substance abuse is common. Examples of remedies for this miasm are *Syphilinum, Mercurius vivus,* and *Aurum metallicum.*

Other miasms have been described more recently, including "Tubercular," "Cancer," "Acute," "Ringworm," and "Rabies."

The idea of miasms is often useful in case analysis. This idea seldom leads to a correct prescription in itself, but may help narrow the field of remedies.

Here is a case example. J.N. is a forty-five-year-old male who comes to see me because he is acutely suicidal (2–3). He is a social worker and was in good health until the last three weeks. One of his teenage patients accused him of sexually molesting her three weeks ago (she would later retract this and state that she had been lying). There is an investigation going on that is very much in the public eye. He immediately felt tremendous grief (3), rage (3), and mortification (3), even though he was innocent. He has to exercise for three hours a day to control his anger (3). He has had thoughts of driving off a cliff (2) or shooting himself with a gun (2). There is a very strong family history of depression (3). His father, grandfather, and great grandfather all committed suicide and had recurrent problems with depression. His depression is worse at night (2). He describes this experience as "eating away at my soul like a malignant ulcer."

The miasm in this case is syphilitic. Syphilitic remedies can be found in the rubric in the Generalities section (1406). I chose *Aurum metallicum*, as it is a syphilitic remedy that is very sensitive to grief, mortification, with feelings of rage, and suicidal depression, especially with thoughts of going over a cliff. He was given a single dosage of *Aurum metallicum* 1M and improved immediately. Within seventy-two hours he was feeling much better with no further suicidal ideation or anger. He continued to do quite well after that, with no recurrence of symptoms.

Taking the Case of the Family

Sometimes individuals need the same remedy that their parents or relatives need. This is especially true in infants and small children. When you can't find the right remedy for the child, taking the case of the parent whom the child most resemble can be helpful. Taking the case of the child may help you find the right remedy for the parent as well.

M.C. is an eighteen-month-old girl. She has had an ear infection for three days (2). There are few symptoms other than her pulling at her right ear (1), a consistent fever of 101 degrees, and irritability (2). She also has no appetite (2). Her mother is breast-feeding her. Her mother feels generally well in the last few days, but notes that she has developed a strong craving for soft-boiled eggs (3) and has been perspiring heavily on the back of her neck during sleep (2) in the last three days.

The symptoms of the ear infection are common and not particularly useful in finding the remedy. However, the mother's symptoms of craving eggs (485) and perspiration of the scalp at night (222) are quite strong and characteristic of the remedy *Calcarea carbonica*. The child was given *Calcarea carbonica* 30C and the symptoms resolved completely in six hours. Interestingly, the mother's cravings for eggs and perspiration at night also resolved quickly.

Chaotic Cases

Sometimes cases are quite unclear and disordered. This can happen when there have been many previous homeopathic prescriptions, allopathic prescriptions or the usage of combination homeopathic remedies in the past. When this occurs, the best strategy is to wait until the case becomes more clear. This can take some time.

Very rarely, you may need to give a remedy to help clear the case. Remedies such as *Sulphur*, *Sepia* or *Nux vomica* have been used for this purpose in the past. Another strategy is to give the closest nosode. For example, if an individual has characteristics that most strongly indicate the sycotic miasm and there is a sycotic family history, then you might give the remedy *Medorrhinum*. Once this remedy has been given, then you need to reevaluate the case as it becomes more clear and find the correct remedy.

Combinations

The best results are obtained when a variety of analysis strategies all confirm the same remedy. When the essence of a case, the totality of symptoms, and the characteristic symptoms all confirm the same remedy, you can prescribe that remedy with great confidence. Unfortunately, this seldom happens. When a prescription is confirmed by a combination of essence and totality, essence and characteristic symptoms, or totality and characteristic symptoms, you can prescribe that remedy with good confidence. Some cases, however, due to suppression, a weak vital force, or lack of homeopathic knowledge, are unclear. This is when imagination, perception, and deep study are the keys to unlocking the heart of the case.

Notes for Lesson Ten

Quiz for Lesson Ten

1. Which of the following is the most true of the Doctrine of Signatures?

    A. A concept first described by Samuel Hahnemann
    B. Represents the characteristic properties of a family of remedies
    C. Represents an integral part of the concept of miasm
    D. Represents the similarity between the properties of a substance and what it heals
    E. Represents the characteristic symptom that best describes a particular remedy

2. Which of the following miasms is best represented by the following three symptoms: "Feels better at night," "severe vaginal discharge," "warts."

    A. Psoric Miasm
    B. Tubercular miasm
    C. Sycotic Miasm
    D. Syphilitic Miasm

3. Which kingdom of remedies best represents the following want ad? "I am a sensitive romantic woman who enjoys nature, music, and art. Let me nurture you."

    A. Imponderables
    B. Plants
    C. Animals
    D. Minerals

4. Which of the following would not be a characteristic symptom in a case?

    A. Throat pain better when swallowing solids
    B. Shoulder pain as if it were being torn off at the socket
    C. Right ear pain during an ear infection
    D. Burning pain in the feet at 3:30 a.m. every night
    E. Numbness of the nose alternating with diarrhea

5. Which remedies are most helpful in clearing chaotic cases?

    A. *Sepia, Calcarea carbonica, Sulphur*
    B. *Sepia, Calcarea carbonica, Rhus toxicodendron*
    C. *Sulphur, Lycopodium clavatum, Calcarea carbonica*
    D. *Sepia, Nux vomica, Sulphur*
    E. *Bryonia alba, Nux vomica, Sulphur*

6. Which of the following case analysis strategies would you first consider for this case?

   L.P. is a fifteen-year-old female with influenza. She has had this for five days. She has had a fever of 102 degrees. She has an occipital headache (1), sore throat (2), and a mild cough (2). There are swollen lymph nodes on both sides of the neck. She is thirsty (1–2). She has had severe low back pain alternating with diarrhea for three days (2–3).

   A. Essence
   B. Totality
   C. Characteristic Symptoms
   D. Doctrine of Signatures
   E. Family/Kingdom

7. Which of the following case analysis strategies would you first consider for this case?

   N.D. is a twenty-eight-year-old year male who has had severe gastritis (3) for one week. This started after he was fired suddenly and without warning from his job. The pain is worse after eating (2) and is burning in character (2). He is worse after eating spicy foods and drinking coffee (1). He is worse when lying down at night and better sitting up (1–2).

   A. Essence
   B. Totality
   C. Characteristic Symptoms
   D. Etiology
   E. Pathology

8. Which of the following case analysis strategies would you first consider for this case?

   M.Z. is a fifty-six-year-old female who was in a car accident five days ago and has been in a coma ever since. She was in good health prior to the accident. She is unresponsive on examination, but nothing else of significance was noted.

   A. Essence
   B. Totality
   C. Characteristic Symptoms
   D. Etiology
   E. Pathology

Practice Cases

Below you will find ten practice cases. Study each case and consider what is most important and characteristic about each case. Try to repertorize the symptoms that are most important. Finally, try to choose the best possible remedy(s) for each case. Answers are found in Appendix L.

Case #1

J.P. is a forty-seven-year-old male. He stepped on a rusty nail on the sole of his foot several days ago. It is moderately swollen (2) and quite painful (2). He describes a pain like a sharp splinter. The wound looks bluish with bruising (2), and there is no drainage. He describes his foot as being colder than normal (1). He finds that the wound feels better with ice packs (2).

Case #2

M.C. is a twenty-five-year-old woman. She calls me in much distress due to urinary pain (3). This started very suddenly four hours ago. She has a long history of urinary tract infections in the past. She describes the pain in the bladder as violent (3). The pain is fairly constant, and described as burning (3) and worse when she urinates. There is much tenesmus (cramping) (2). She's passing large clots of blood (2). She is feeling quite irritable (2), anxious (2), and restless (2). She describes no particular causation.

Case #3

You do a visit on a sixty-seven-year-old female with severe chronic shortness of breath who is housebound and on oxygen. She has chronic bronchitis, which seems to come on every winter (2). She has developed bronchitis again in the last five days (3). She is breathing poorly and is quite blue (2). There is much rattling of mucus in her chest (3), and she is having great difficulty getting up the mucus. She lacks the energy to rise to greet you. She is better when sitting up (2). She is worse when in a warm room and worse when lying down. There is swelling of the legs (2) and drowsiness (2).

Case #4

P.R. is a five year old female with a cough related to croup that has been going on for ten days. It is nonproductive (dry). It sounds like a seal barking (croupy cough) (2). It is worse in late evening (from nine to eleven p.m.) (2). It is better when drinking hot tea (2) and worse when drinking cold fluids (3). There is hoarseness (2). The throat is painful (1–2) and worse after coughing (2). She is quite anxious and fearful (2). She is thirstier than usual. Her cervical (neck) glands are swollen and tender (2).

Case #5

C.Z. is a fifty-five-year-old woman who has had severe headaches (3) for the last several months following whiplash in a car accident. The headaches start in the neck and radiate over the top of the head to the forehead (3). They are associated with dizziness and a feeling of falling (2). They are worse in the morning, especially between nine and eleven a.m. The head feels like a band around the forehead (2). The scalp is sore to the touch (1). The neck feels weak (1). She feels quite dull (2) and depressed (1). She has noticed a tremor of her hands since the accident. She is having difficulty sleeping (2); once she is awoken, she cannot fall back to sleep again. There is mild blurred vision, and her vision is especially a problem at night when she is driving (2). She has not been hungry or thirsty since the accident and has lost fifteen pounds. She has been craving sweets (1) when she does eat.

Case #6

J.M. is a twenty-seven-year-old male who has influenza. This started three days ago and has gotten steadily worse. He had been out working in the yard in rainy weather the day before it began. It started with a sore throat that has also gotten progressively worse (2). The sore throat is better with warm drinks (2). He becomes hoarse when he first starts talking, but then the hoarseness dissipates after he talks for a while (1–2). He is quite chilly (2). There is aching in all the joints (2). This is especially true in the lower back (3). He is quite restless and unable to keep still (2). He desires cold drinks (2) and sweets (1). He is sleeping poorly. There is no fever.

Case #7

C.S. is a fourteen-year-old girl who has severe dysmenorrhea (3). The pain is most-ly left-sided (2) and crampy in nature (2). She is unable to attend school for several days prior to her period. She experiences simultaneously diarrhea and vomiting (2) during that time, coupled with profuse perspiration (2) and great chilliness

(3). The symptoms are worse in the morning (2). She has problems with icy cold hands, which turn blue (2) (Raynaud's Syndrome). There are cravings for sweets (2), salt (3) and fruit (2). Palpitations of the chest are often associated (1).

Case #8

J.C. is an eighteen-year-old female who is quite ill with influenza. This started several days ago, and she has become progressively more ill. She is very sleepy (2–3) and confused (2). She falls asleep when she is talking to you. Her temperature is 103.5 degrees. She complains of a mild sore throat, which has a deep red color (2) on examination. She is having trouble swallowing; this is worse when swallowing solids (1–2). She complains of feeling sore and stiff all over (2) and cannot find a comfortable position in bed. Her mouth has a very foul odor (3). She is craving salt (1) and lemonade (1). She is perspiring heavily and there is mild diarrhea. She says that her dreams are quite busy (2). Her face is red (2).

Case #9

J.T. is a five-year-old boy with an acute right-sided ear infection that started yesterday in his sleep. The ear infection started after his brother broke his favorite toy. He is screaming (2) from the pain and won't let you examine his ear. The ear drum looks very red and swollen. His mother cannot satisfy him (2), and he keeps changing his mind about what he wants (2). He does not want to be touched (2). His mother notes that he cried in his sleep last night (2–3). He also has diarrhea and has loose green stools (1–2).

Case #10

P.K. is a seven-year-old female who has developed acute bronchitis associated with asthma (2) over the last three days. She is irritable. She complains of severe headaches (2). She has been craving cold drinks (2). She has been nauseous (3) and cannot stop vomiting (3). She has been unable to keep any food down. There has been some blood with the expectoration (1). She complains of feeling hotter than usual. She has abdominal pain and discomfort (1–2).

APPENDICES

APPENDIX A

Acute Casetaking Template

Name _____

Address _____

Phone _____

Age _____

Sex _____

Chief Complaint: _____ X _____ weeks

    Modalities:

    Concomitants:

    Description in Detail:

    Onset:

Temperature:

GI: Desires   Aversions   Thirst

Perspiration:

Mentals:

Sleep:

Generalities:

Past Medical History (if appropriate):

Physical Examination:

Impression:

Plan: (Include when to follow up and return)

APPENDIX B

Sample Review of Systems Questionnaire

If you have been bothered *recently* by any of these problems check yes:

Y	N		Y	N		Y	N	
☐	☐	frequent/severe headaches	☐	☐	pain in abdomen	☐	☐	family problems
☐	☐	back pains	☐	☐	bloated abdomen	☐	☐	problems at work
☐	☐	neck lumps or swelling	☐	☐	constipation	☐	☐	sexual difficulties
☐	☐	loss of balance	☐	☐	loose bowels	☐	☐	change of sexual energy
☐	☐	dizzy spells	☐	☐	black stools	☐	☐	considered suicide
☐	☐	blackouts/fainting	☐	☐	grey or whitish stools	☐	☐	loss or gain in weight
☐	☐	wear glasses	☐	☐	pain in rectum	☐	☐	loss of appetite
☐	☐	blurry vision	☐	☐	Itching rectum	☐	☐	always hungry
☐	☐	eyesight worsening	☐	☐	blood with stools	☐	☐	fatigue or weariness
☐	☐	see double	☐	☐	frequent urination	☐	☐	fever or chills
☐	☐	see halos or lights	☐	☐	involuntary urination	☐	☐	motion sickness
☐	☐	eye pains or itching	☐	☐	burning on urination	☐	☐	night sweats
☐	☐	watering eyes	☐	☐	black or bloody urine	☐	☐	hot flashes
☐	☐	earaches	☐	☐	weak urine stream	☐	☐	warm or cold than others
☐	☐	hearing difficulties	☐	☐	difficulty starting urine			
☐	☐	running ears	☐	☐	constant urge to urinate			**Men Only**
☐	☐	noises in ears	☐	☐	aching muscles or joints	☐	☐	burning or discharge
☐	☐	dental problems	☐	☐	swollen joints	☐	☐	swelling on testicles
☐	☐	sore or bleeding gums	☐	☐	back or shoulder pains	☐	☐	painful testicles
☐	☐	sore tongue	☐	☐	weakness in arms/legs			
☐	☐	congested nose	☐	☐	painful feet			**Women Only**
☐	☐	running nose	☐	☐	trembling	☐	☐	missed period
☐	☐	sneezing spells	☐	☐	numbness	☐	☐	menstrual problems
☐	☐	head colds	☐	☐	leg cramps	☐	☐	bleeding between periods
☐	☐	nosebleeds	☐	☐	skin problems	☐	☐	heavy bleeding
☐	☐	sore throat	☐	☐	scalp problems	☐	☐	bearing down feeling
☐	☐	difficulty swallowing	☐	☐	itching or burning skin	☐	☐	vaginal discharge
☐	☐	hoarse voice	☐	☐	bruise easily	☐	☐	genital irritation
☐	☐	wheezing or gasping	☐	☐	nervousness or anxiety	☐	☐	pain on intercourse
☐	☐	frequent coughing	☐	☐	nervous with strangers	☐	☐	swelling of breasts
☐	☐	cough up phlegm	☐	☐	nail biting	☐	☐	# of pregnancies
☐	☐	cough up blood	☐	☐	difficulty making decisions	☐	☐	# of births
☐	☐	chest colds	☐	☐	lack of concentration	_____		# of miscarriages
☐	☐	rapid or skipped heart beats	☐	☐	loss of memory	_____		# of premature births
☐	☐	chest pains	☐	☐	lonely or depressed	_____		# of caesarean
☐	☐	shortness of breath	☐	☐	frequent crying	_____		# of abortions
☐	☐	swollen feet or ankles	☐	☐	hopeless outlook			
☐	☐	armpits or groin swelling	☐	☐	difficulty relaxing			Comments or special problems:
☐	☐	difficulty sleeping	☐	☐	worry a lot			
☐	☐	motion sickness	☐	☐	scary dreams or thoughts			
☐	☐	excessive sweating	☐	☐	feeling of desperation			
☐	☐	recurring indigestion	☐	☐	shy or sensitive			
☐	☐	frequent belching	☐	☐	dislike criticism			
☐	☐	nausea	☐	☐	angered easily			
☐	☐	vomiting	☐	☐	annoyed by little things			

Sample Family History Questionnaire

Place an (X) in the appropriate column for any illness that you or your relatives have had.

ILLNESS	Self	Father	Mother	Brothers	Sisters	Child #1	Child #2	Child #3	Grandparents
Abnormal Periods									
Alcohol/Drugs									
Allergies									
Anemia									
Arthritis/Gout									
Asthma									
Bleeding Problems									
Cancer									
Diabetes									
Eczema									
Emphysema									
Epilepsy									
Frequent Infections									
Heart Trouble									
Hepatitis									
High Blood Pressure									
Kidney Problems									
Mental Illness									
Migraines									
Polio									
Pneumonia									
Prostrate Problems									
Psoriasis									
Rheumatic Fever									
Stomach Problems									
Stroke									
Thyroid Problems									
Tuberculosis									
Ulcers									
Venereal Disease									
Weight Problems									

Remedies and Their Abbreviations in Kent's Repertory

Abies-c: Abies canadensis

Abies-n: Abies nigra

Abrot: Abrotanum

Absin: Absinthum

Acal: Acalypha indica

Acet-ac: Acetic acid

Acon-c: Aconitum cammarum

Acon: Aconitum napellus

Acon-f: Aconitum ferox

Acon-i: Aconitum lycotonum

Act-sp: Actea spicata

Aesc: Aesculus hippocastanum

Aesc-g: Aesculus glabra

Aeth: Aethusa cyapium

Agar-em: Agaricus emeticus

Agar: Agaricus muscarius

Agar-ph: Agaricus phalloides

Agn: Agnus castus

Ail: Ailanthus

Alco: Alcohol

Alet: Aletris farinosa

All-c: Allium cepa

All-s: Allium sativum

Aloe: Aloe scotrina

Alst: Alstonia constricta

Alumn: Alumen

Alum: Alumina

Alum-m: Alumina metallicum

Alum-sil: Alumina silicata

Ambr: Ambra Grisea

Ambro: Ambrosia artemisiae folia

Ammc: Ammoniacum bummi

Am-be: Ammonium benzoicum

Am-br: Ammonium bromatum

Am-c: Ammonium carbonicum

Am-caust: Ammonium causticum

Am-m: Ammonium muriaticum

Amph: Amphisboena

Amyg: Amygdalae amarae aqua

Aml-n: Amyl nitrite

Anac: Anacardium orientale

Anac-oc: Acacardium occidentale

Anag: Anagallis arvensis

Anan: Anantherum muricatum

Ang: Angustra Vera

Anil: Anilinum

Anis: Anisum stellatum

Anth: Anthemis nobilis

Anthr: Anthracinum

Anthro: Anthrokokali

Ant-a: Antimonium arsenicosum

Ant-c: Antimonium crudum

Ant-chl: Antimonium cholidum

Ant-ox: Antimonium oxydatum

Ant-s: Antimonium sulfa, erratum

Ant-t: Antimonium tartaricum

Aphis: Aphis chenopodii glauci

Apis: Apis mellifica

Ap-g: Apium graveolens

Apoc: Apocynum cannabinum

Apoc-a: Apocynum androsa-emifolium

Apom: Apomorphium

Aral: Aralia racemosa

Aran: Aranea diadema

Aran-s: Aranea sciencia

Arg-c: Argentum cyanidum

Arg-m: Argentum metallicum

Arg-mur: Argentum muriaticum

Arg-n: Argentum nitricum

Arn: Arnica montana

Ars: Arsenicum album

Ars-h: Arsenicum hydrogenesiatum

Ars-i: Arsenicum iodatum

Ars-m: Arsenicum metallicum

Ars-s-f: Arsenicum sulphuratum flavum

Ars-s-r: Arsencium sulphuratum rubrum

Art-v: Artemisia vulgaris

Arum-d: Arum draconitum

Arum-i: Arum italicum

Arum-t: Arum triphyllum

Arun: Arundo mauritianica

Arund-d: Arundo donna

Asaf: Asafoetida

Asar: Asarum europaeum

Asc-c: Asclepias tuberosa

Asim: Asimina tribloba

Aspar: Asparagus officinalis

Astac: Astacus fluvialis

Atro: Atropinum

Atro-s: Atrophia sulphurica

Aur: Aurum metallicum

Aur-a: Aurum arsenicosum

Aur-i: Aurum iodatum

Aur-m: Aurum muriaticum

Aur-m-n: Aurum muriaticum natronatum

Aur-s: Aurum sulphuricum

Bad: Badiaga

Bals: Balsamum peruvianum

Bapt: Baptisia tintoria

Bart: Bartfelder (acid spring)

Bar-ac: Baryta acetica

Bar-c: Baryta carbonica

Bar-i: Baryta iodatum

Bar-m: Baryta muriatica

Bell: Belladonna

Bell-p: Bellis perennis

Benz: Benzinum

Benz-ac: Benzoic acidum

Benz-n: Benzinum nitricum

Berb: Berberis vulgaris

Bism: Bismuthum oxidum

Blat: Blatta americana

Blatta: Blatta orientalis

Bol: Boletus laricis

Bor-ac: Boracicum acidum

Bor: Borax

Both: Bothrops lanceolatus

Bov: Bovista

Brach: Brachyglottis repens

Brom: Bromium
Brac: Bracea antidsenterica
Bry: Bryonia alba
Bufo: Bufo rana
Bufo-s: Bufo sahytiensis
Cact: Cactus grandiflorux
Cadm: Cadmium sulphuratum
Cahin: Cahinca
Cain: Cainca
Caj: Cajuputum
Calad: Caladium seguinum
Calc-ac: Calcarea acetica
Calc-ar: Calcarea arsenica
Calc: Calcarea carbonica
Calc-caust: Calcarea caustica
Calc-f: Calcarea flourica
Calc-i: Calcarea iodata
Calc-p: Calcarea phosphorica
Calc-sil: Calcarea silicata
Calc-s: Calcarea sulphurica
Calen: Calendula officinalis
Calli: Calliandra houstoni
Calo: Calotropis gigantea
Calt: Caltha palustris
Camph: Camphora officinarum
Canch: Canchalugua
Cann-i: Cannabis indica
Cann-s: Cannabis sativa
Canth: Cantharis
Caps: Capsicum
Carb-ac: Carbolic acidum
Carb-an: Carbo animalis
Carb-h: Carboneum hydro-
    genesiatum
Carbo-o: Carboneum oxygenisatum
Carb-s: Carboneum sulphuratum
Carb-v: Carbo vegetabilis
Card-b: Carduus benedictus
Card-m: Carduus marianus
Carl: Carlsbad
Casc: Cascarilla
Cast-v: Castanea vesca
Cas-eq: Castor equi
Cast: Castoreum
Caul: Caulophyllum thalictroides
Caust: Causticum
Cean: Ceanothus americanus
Cedr: Cedron
Cench: Cenchris contortirx
Cent: Centaurea tagana
Cere-b: Cereus bonplandii

Cer-s: Cereux serpentaria
Cet: Cetrararia islandica
Cham: Chamomilla
Chel: Chelidonium majus
Chen-a: Chenoopodium
    anthelminticum
Chen-v: Chenopodium vulvaria
Chim: Chimaphilia umbellata
Chim-m: Chimaphilia maculata
Chin: China officinalis
Chin-a: Chininum arsenicosum
Chin-b: China boliviana
Chin-s: Chininum sulphuricum
Chion: Chionanthus virginica
Chlol: Chloralum
Chlf: Chloroform
Chlor: Chlorum
Chol: Cholesterinum
Chr-as: Chromic acidum
Chr-ox: Chromic acidum
Cic: Cicuta virosa
Cimex: Cimex
Cimic: Cimicifuga racemosa
Cina: Cina
Cinnb: Cinnabaris
Cinnam: Cinnamomum ceylanicum
Cist: Cistus canadensis
Cit-ac: Citric acid
Cit-l: Citrus limonum
Cit-v: Citrus vulgaris
Clem: Clematis erecta
Cob: Cobaltum
Coca: Coca
Cocaine: Cocainum muriaticum
Cocc: Cocculus indica
Cocc-t: Coccinella septempuncata
Cocc-c: Coccus cacti
Coch: Cochleria armoracia
Cod: Codeinum
Coff: Coffea cruda
Coff-t: Coffea tosta
Colch: Colchicum autumnale
Coll : Collinsonia canadensis
Coloc: Colocynthis
Colos: Colustrum
Com: Comocladia dentata
Con: Conium maculatum
Conv: Convallaria majalis
Conv-d: Convolvulus duartinus
Cop: Copaiva officinalis
Cor-r: Corallium rubrum

Cori-r: Coriaria rusicifolia
Corn: Cornus circinata
Cornus-f: Cornus florida
Cornus-s: Cornus serica
Croc: Crocus sativus
Cot: Cotyledon umbilicius
Crot-c: Crotalus cascavella
Crot-h: Crotalus horridus
Crot-t: Croton tiglium
Cub: Cubeba officinalis
Culx: Culex moscae
Cund: Cundurango
Cupr: Cuprum Metallicum
Cupr-a: Cuprum aceticum
Cupr-ar: Cuprum arsenicosum
Cupr-n: Cuprum nitricum
Cupr-s: Cuprum sulphuricum
Cur: Curare
Cycl: Cyclamen eurpaecum
Cyp: Cypripedium pubescens
Daph: Daphne indica
Der : Derris pinnata
Dig: Digitalis purpurea
Dios : Dioscorea villosa
Dol: Dolichos pruriens
Dor: Doryphora
Dros: Drosera rotundifolia
Dub: Duboisinum
Dul: Dulcamara
Echi: Echinacea angustifolia
Elaps: Elaps carallinus
Elat: Elaterium officinarum
Epig: Egige repens
Equis: Equisetum hyernale
Erech: Erechthites hieracifolia
Erighi: Erigeron canadense
Ery-a: Eryngium aquaticum
Ether: Ether
Eucal: Eucalyptus globulus
Eug: Eugeneia jambos
Euon: Euonyumus europaeus
Eup-per: Eupatorium perfoliatum
Eup-pur: Eupatorium purpureum
Euph: Euphorbium
Euphr: Euphrasia officinalis
Eupi: Eupion
Fago: Fagopyrum
Ferr-ar: Ferrum arsenicosum
Ferr: Ferrum metallicum
Ferr-ac: Ferrum aceticum
Ferr-i: Ferrum iodatum

Ferr-ma: Ferrum magneticum

Ferr-p: Ferrum phosphoricum

Ferr-pic: Ferrum picricum

Ferr-s: Ferrum sulphuricum

Fil: Filix max

Fl-ac: Floricum acidum

Form: Formica rufa

Frag-v: Fragaria vesca

Gad: Gadus morrhua

Gall-ac: Gallicum acidum

Gamb: Gambogia

Gels: Gelsemium sempervirens

Genist: Genista tintoria

Gent-l: Gentiana lutea

Gent-c: Gentiana cruciata

Ger: Germanium maculatum

Get: Gettisburg water

Gins: Ginseng

Gland: Glanderine

Glon: Glonoinum

Gnaph: Gnaphalium

Goss: Gossypium heraceum

Gran: Granatum punica

Graph: Graphites

Grat: Gratiola officinalis

Grin: Grindelia robusta

Gua: Guaco

Guano: Guano aust

Guar: Guarana

Guare: Guarca

Guaj: Guiacum

Gymn: Gymnocladus

Ham: Hamamelis virginica

Hecla: Hecla lava

Hedeom: Hedeoma pulegioides

Hell: Helleborus niger

Helo: Heloderma

Helon: Helonias dioica

Hep: Hepar sulphuris calcareum

Hipp: Hippomanes

Hippoz: Hiipozaenium

Hom: Homarus

Hur: Hura braziliensis

Hydrang: Hydrangea arborescens

Hydrc: Hydrocotyle asiatica

Hydr-ac: Hydrocyanic acid

Hyos: Hyoscyamus niger

Hyper: Hypericum perforatum

Iber: Iberis amara

Ictod: Ictodes foetida

Ign: Ignatia amara

Ill: Illicium anisatum

Ind: Indigo

Ing: Ingluvin

Inul: Inula helenium

Iodof: Iodoforum

Iod: Iodium

Ip: Ipecacuanha

Ipom: Ipomia purpurea

Iridium: Iridium

Ir-fl: Iris florentina

Ir-foe: Iris foetidissima

Ir-g: Iris germanica

Iris: Iris versicolor

Jab: Jaborandi

Jac: Jacaranda gualandai

Jac-c: Jacaranda caroba

Jal: Jalapa

Jatr: Jatropha curcas

Jug-c: Juglans cinerea

Jug-r: Juglans regia

Junc: Juncus effusus

Juni: Juniperus verginiana

Kali-a: Kali aceticum

Kali-ar: Kali arsenicosum

Kali-bi: Kali bichromicum

Kali-br: Kali bromatum

Kali-c: Kali carbonicum

Kali-chl: Kali chloricum

Kali-cy: Kali cyanatum

Kali-fer: Kali ferrocyanium

Kali-i: Kali iodatum

Kali-m: Kali muriaticum

Kali-ma: Kali manganicum

Kali-n: Kali nitricum

Kali-ox: Kali oxalicum

Kali-p: Kali phosphoricum

Kali-s: Kali sulphuricum

Kalm: Kalmia latifolia

Kaol: Kaolin

Kino: Kino

Kiss: Kissengen

Kreos: Kreosotum

Lac-c: Lac caninum

Lac-d: Lac defloratum

Lac-f: Lac felinum

Lach: Lachesis

Lachn: Lachnanthes tinctoria

Lac-ac: Lactic acid

Lact: Lactuca virosa

Lam: Lamium album

Lap-a: Lapis albus

Lapp-a: Lappa articum

Lapp-m: Lappa major

Lath: Lathyrus sativus

Lat-m: Latrodectus mactans

Laur: Lauroceraseus

Lec: Lecithinum

Led: Ledum palustre

Lem-m: Lemna minor

Lepi: Lepidium bonariense

Lept: Leptandra virginica

Lil-t: Lilium tigrinum

Linu-c: Linum cathar

Lith: Lithium carbonicum

Lith-m: Lithium muriaticum

Lob-c: Lobelia cardinalis

Lob: Lobelia inflata

Lob-s: Lobelia syphilitica

Lup: Lupulus

Lyc: Lycopodium clavatum

Lycpr: Lycopersicum esculentum

Lycps: Lycopus virginicus

Lyss: Lyssinum (Hydrophobinum)

Mag-arct: Magnetis polus arcticus

Mag-asut: Magnetis polus australis

Mag-c: Magnesia carbonica

Mag-m: Magnesia muriatica

Mag-p: Magnesia phosphorica

Mag-p-s: Magnetis pulus ambo

Mag-s: Magnesia sulphurica

Maland: Malandrium

Malar: Malaria officinalis

Manc: Mancinella (Hippomanes)

Mang: Manganum

Mang-m: Manganum muriaticum

Med: Medorrhinum

Meli: Melilotus alba

Menis: Menispermum

Ment: Metha piperita

Meny: Menyanthes

Meph: Mephites

Merc: Mercurius vivus (dulcis)

Merc-ac: Mercurius aceticus

Merc-c: Mercurius corrosivus

Merc-cy: Mercurius cyanatus

Merc-i-f: Mercurius iodatus flavus

Merc-i-r: Mercurius iodatus ruber

Merc-n: Mercurius nitrosus

Merc-p-r: Mercurius praecipitatus ruber

Merc-sul: Mercurium sulphuratum

Merl: Mercurialis perennis

Mez: Mezereum

Mill: Millefolium
Mit: Mitchella repens
Morph: Morphinum
Mosc: Moschus
Murx: Murex
Mur-ac: Muriatic acidum
Mygal: Mygale lasiodora
Myos: Myosotis
Myric: Myrica cerifera
Myris: Myristica sebifera
Myrt-c: Myrtis communis
Naja: Naja tripudia
Napht: Naphtha
Narcot: Narcotinum
Nat-ac: Natrum aceticum
Nat-a: Natrum arsenicosum
Nat-c: Natrum carbonicum
Nat-h: Natrum hypochlorosum
Nat-m: Natrum muriaticum
Nat-n: Natrum nitricum
Nat-p: Natrum phosphoricum
Nat-s: Natrum sulphuricum
Nicc: Niccolum
Nicc-s: Niccolum sulphuricum
Nit-ac: Nitric acidum
Nit-m-ac: Nitris spiriti dulcis
Nitro-o: Nitrogenum oxygenatum
Nuph: Nuphar luteum
Nux-m: Nux moschata
Nux-j: Nux juglans
Nux-v: Nux vomica
Nym: Nymphea odorata
Oci: Ocimum canum
Oena: Oenanthe crocata
Olnd: Oleander
Ol-an: Oleum animale
Ol-j: Oleum jecoris aselli
Onos: Onosmodium
Op: Opium
Orig: Origanum majorana
Osm: Osmium
Ov: Ovinine
Ox-ac: Oxalic acidum
Oxyt: Oxytropis lamberti
Ozone: Ozone
Paeon: Paeonia officinalis
Pall: Palladium
Pareir: Pareira brava
Par: Paris quadrifolia
Paull: Paullinia pinnata
Ped: Pediculus capitis

Pen: Penthorum
Per: Persica
Peti: Petiveria
Petr: Petroleum
Petros: Petroselinum
Phal: Phallus impudicum
Phase : Phaseolus nanum
Phel: Phellandium
Ph-ac: Phosphoric acidum
Phos: Phosphorous
Phys: Physogstigma
Phyt: Phytolacca decandra
Pic-ac: Picric acid
Pimp: Pimpinella saxifraga
Pinus-s: Pinus sylvestris
Pip-s: Piper methysticum
Pip-n: Piper nigrum
Plan: Plantago major
Plat: Platinum metallicum
Plat-m: Platinum muriaticum
Plect: Plectranthus
Plumbg: Plumbago littoralis
Plb: Plumbum metallicum
Popd: Podophyllum peltatum
Polg: Polygonum hydropiperoides
Pop: Populus tremuloides
Poth: Pothos foetidus
Prun: Prunus spinosa
Psor: Psorinum
Ptel: Ptelea trifoliata
Pulx: Pulex iritans
Puls: Pulsatilla nigricans
Pul-n: Pulsatilla nuttaliana
Pyrog: Pyrogenium
Pyrus: Pyrus americana
Rad: Radium
Ran-a: Ranunculus acris
Ran-b: Ranunculus bulbosus
Ran-s: Ranunculus scleratus
Raph: Raphanus
Rat: Ratanhia
Rheum: Rheum
Rhod: Rhododendron
Rhus-a: Rhus aromatica
Rhus-g: Rhus glabra
Rhus-r: Rhus radicans
Rhus-t: Rhus toxicodendron
Rhus-v: Rhus venanata
Rob: Robinia pseudacacia
Rumex: Rumex crispus
Ruta: Ruta graveolens

Sabad: Sabadilla
Sabal: Sabal serrulata
Sabin: Sabina
Sacc: Saccharum album
Sac-l: Saccharum lactis
Sal-ac: Salicylicum acidum
Salam: Salamander
Sal-n: Salix niger
Samb: Sambucus nigra
Sang: Sanguinaria canadensis
Sang-n: Sanguinaria nitrica
Sanic: Sanicula aqua
Sant: Santoninum
Sarr: Sarracenia purpurea
Sars: Sarsasparilla
Scut: Scutellaria lateriflora
Sec: Secale cornutum
Sel: Selenium
Senec: Seniecio aureus
Seneg: Senega
Senn: Senna
Sep: Sepia
Serp: Serpentaria
Sil: Silicaea
Sin-a: Sinapsis alba
Sin-n: Sinapsis nigra
Sol-m: Solanum mammosum
Sol-n: Solanum nigrum
Sol-o: Solanum oleraceum
Sol-t-ae: Solanum tuberosum aegrotans
Sol-v: Solidago virgaurea
Spig: Spigelia anthelmia
Spig-m: Spigelia marilandica
Spira: Spiranthes
Spong: Spongia tosta
Squil: Squilla hispanica
Stach: Stachya betonica
Staph: Staphysagria
Stel: Stellaria media
Stict: Sticta pulmonaria
Still: Stillangia sylvatica
Stram: Stramonium
Stront: Strontium
Strop: Strophanthus hispidus
Stry: Strychninum
Sulph: Sulphur
Sul-i: Sulphur iodatum
Sul-ac: Sulphuric acidum
Sumb: Sumbul
Syph: Syphilinum
Symph: Symphytum officinale

Sym-r: Symphoricarpus racemosus
Tab: Tabacum
Tanac: Tanacetum vulgare
Tann: Tanninum
Tarax: Taraxicum
Tarent: Tarentula hispanica
Tarent-c: Tarentula cubensis
Tart-ac: Tartaric acidum
Tax: Taxus baccata
Tel: Tellurium
Tep : Teplitz aqua
Ter: Terebinthina
Teucr: Teucrium marum verum
Thal: Thallium
Thea: Thea sinensis
Ther: Theridion
Thlaspi: Thlaspi bursa pastoris
Thuja : Thuja occidentalis
Til: Tilia europoea
Tong: Tongo

Trif-p: Trifolium patense
Tril: Trilium pendulum
Trom: Trombidium muscae domesticae
Trio: Triosteum perfoliatum
Tub: Tuberculinum
Tus-f: Tussilago fragrans
Tus-p: Tussilago petasites
Upa: Upas tiente
Uran: Uranium nitricum
Urt-u: Urtica urens
Ust: Ustilago maydis
Uva: Uva ursi
Vac: Vaccinotoxinum
Valer: Valeriana
Vario: Variolinum
Verat: Veratrum album
Verat-v: Veratrum viride
Verb: Verbascum thapsus
Vesp: Vespa crabro

Vib: Viburnum opulus
Vinc: Vinca minor
Viol-o: Viola odorata
Viol-t: Viola tricolorata
Vip: Vipera
Visc: Viscum album
Wies: Wiesbaden aqua
Wild: Wildbad aqua
Wye: Wyethia helenioides
Xan: Xanthoxylum fraxineum
Yuc: Yucca
Zinc: Zincum metallicum
Zinc-ac: Zincum aceticum
Zinc-c: Zincum cyanatum
Zinc-m: Zincum muriaticum
Zinc-ox: Zincum oxydatum
Zinc-s: Zincum sulphuricum
Zing: Zingiber
Ziz: Zizia aurea

The sixty most frequent remedies in Kent's repertory are:

1. Sulph
2. Phos
3. Lyc
4. Sep
5. Calc
6. Puls
7. Nat-m
8. Ars
9. Nux-v
10. Merc
11. Rhus-t
12. Sil
13. Bell
14. Lach
15. Thuja
16. Caust
17. Bry
18. Kali Carb
19. Zinc
20. Nit-ac
21. Carb-v
22. Alum
23. Graph
24. Agar
25. Con
26. Chin
27. Hep
28. Ph-ac
29. Acon
30. Nat-c
31. Chel
32. Mez
33. Staph
34. Cham
35. Petr
36. Verat
37. Plb
38. Am-c
39. Arn
40. Kali-bi
41. Bar-c
42. Mag-c
43. Apis
44. Ign
45. Cocc
46. Stram
47. Carb-an
48. Aur
49. Arg-n
50. Ver-alb
51. Coloc
52. Plat
53. Canth
54. Mag-m
55. Berb
56. Iod
57. Spig
58. Nat-s
59. Dulc
60. Hyos

Sections of Kent's Repertory

1. Mind
2. Vertigo
3. Head
4. Eye
5. Vision
6. Ear
7. Hearing
8. Nose
9. Face
10. Mouth
11. Teeth
12. Throat
13. External Throat
14. Stomach
15. Abdomen
16. Rectum
17. Stool
18. Bladder
19. Kidneys
20. Prostate
21. Urethra
22. Urine
23. Male Genitalia
24. Female Genitalia
25. Larynx and Trachea
26. Respiration
27. Cough
28. Expectoration
29. Chest
30. Back
31. Extremities
32. Sleep
33. Chill
34. Fever
35. Perspiration
36. Skin
37. Generalities
38. Index

General Layout of Kent's Repertory

General Rubric
Sidedness Modifiers
Time Modifiers
General Modalities
Extensions
Locations
Descriptor Modifiers

Descriptors of Pain Terminology from the Repertory

Aching: continuous dull pain

Biting: deeper, localized, narrow, sharp form of pinching, severe pinching, kind of localized burning sensation

Blows, as from: sudden impact, large area involved, traumatic sudden impact, jarring, a little confusing, sensation of bruising

Boring, Digging, Screwing: from outside in, working its way in, exact location, steady pain, tight location, mild quality

Burning: hot, red, like fire, more superficial, not confined, blurry edges

Burrowing: tunneling, mild, nagging

Bursting: explosive, splitting, violent, one of the most violent

Come Off, Pains as if Top of Head Would: severe feeling of expansion, not well localized, vibrating

Cramping: on and off in intensity, muscular, superficial, like tied in a knot, griping (more severe form of cramping), nonspecific intensity

Crushed, as if Shattered, Beaten to Pieces: sore, torn, severe, battered, wide distribution

Cutting: sharp, knifelike, intense, extended

Drawing, Tightening: as if something is being pulled from one place to another place, pulling inwards

Dull Pain: mild to moderate intensity, boundaries obscure, constant, not sure when it begins or ends

Foreign Body, as if: sensation of something present that is not normally there

Gnawing: constant, never really gone, intermittent intensity, annoying, weight and pressure, fixed location, chewing

Grasping: constricting, squeezing, pulling, about the size of a hand, digging-in sensation, intermittent, moderate, localized

Grinding: involves motion; wearing smooth by friction or motion

Griping: spasmodic, sudden, hard to ignore, short duration, acute, moderate to severe

Grumbling: turbulence, chronic, annoying, changing but constantly there, easily distracted from, mild to moderate, generalized location

Hacking: cut, notch, slice, chop or severing with heavy irregular like blows

Jerking: pain makes you move, not a pain, its like something that happens in your body, causes movement

Lancinating: jabbing, like a puncture, deeper, big, sharp, penetrating, very painful, stabbing

Nail, as if from a: pointed, sharp, quick and deep, localized

Open, as if Opening and Shutting: involves motion that is repeated

Pecking: quick localizes strokes in a circumscribed area

Pinching: on and off, superficial, tight then lets go, little spots, sting, small localized

Plug, Peg or Wedge, as from a: evolving from a small area to a large area, from the inside to the outside, quite intense, steady, relatively small space, exerts pressure outward from itself

Pressing: wide area, superficial, internal or external, duller, not sharp

Pulled, Sensation as if a Hair Were Pulling: involves movement; see "Drawing"

Shooting: violent, strong, traveling, rapid, traveling is the key

Smarting: sharp, keen, or brisk

Sore, Bruised: general, not deep, only when touched, exacerbated by pressure, not something that hurts unless touched or changed

Stitching: thin, sharp, sudden goes through, well localized, rapid, small, as if drawing something though an area

Stunning, Stupefying: severe, known by the effect it has on you

Tearing: pulling, rough, progressive intensity then diminishes, aware of the progression of the pain, cataclysmic and sudden, clear definition of borders

Throbbing (see Pulsating)

Torn, as if: uneven edges, sharpness, more than one direction to the pain, two distinct places both with pain

Ulcerative: element of burning or stinging, superficial, gnawing, specific location, well-delineated spot, slightly below the surface

Sharp Pains (in order of increasing degree of the pain): 1. Pinching; 2. Biting; 3. Stitching; 4. Shooting; 5. Tearing; 6. Nail, as if from a; 7. Cutting; 8. Lancinating; 9. Bursting

Dull Pains: Blows, as from; Boring, Digging, Screwing; Burning; Burrowing; Come Off, Pain as if Top of Head Would; Cramping; Drawing; Tightening; Dull Pain; Foreign Body, as if; Gnawing; Grasping; Grinding; Griping; Grumbling; Hacking; Pecking; Plug, Peg or Wedge, as from a; Pressing; Pulling; Smarting; Sore, Bruised; Torn, as if

Glossary of Confusing Terminology in the Repertory

Abscess (693): circumscribed collection of pus

Amenorrhea (336): absence of periods

Apoplexy (1176): stroke

Apyrexia During (422): without fever

Areola (992): colored ring

Ascarides (715): roundworms

Atonic (1221): without tone

Atrophy: wasting of tissue

Aura (715): symptom preceding the onset of a seizure

Bifurcation of Trachea (860): part of the windpipe that splits

Blebs (1000): large, soft blisters

Bright's Disease (835): chronic inflammation of the kidneys

Bubo (541): enlarged and infected lymph node

Carbuncle (887): large abscess in which there is a localized collection of pus in a cavity

Caries (108): decay of bone

Catarrh (435): secretion of mucous caused by inflammation related to environmental irritants

Chancres (713): hard ulcers

Cholera (666): bacterial epidemic disease causing profuse watery diarrhea and extreme fluid loss leading to collapse.

Chlorotic (356): pale

Cicatrices (881): scar; normal tissue being replaced by fibrous nonfunctional tissue

Circinate (1312): circular shaped

Climaxis (337): menopause

Clonic (968): alternating contractions and relaxations of muscles

Coitus (849): intercourse

Colliquative (1296): progressive wasting of the body

Collous Edges (1221): gluey

Condylomata (449): warts

Confluent (986): coming together

Congestion (715): full of blood

Crural (1071): large nerve

Cyanotic (359): blueness due to a lack of oxygenation to tissue

Delirium Tremens (1212): form of delirium and psychosis associated with alcohol withdrawal

Desquamation (329): loss or peeling of skin

Dilation (828): enlargement

Dropsy (717): swelling

Dysentery (1308): infectious disease associated with diarrhea and dehydration

Dysmenorrhea (362): pain during menses

Dyspnea With (897): shortness of breath

Ebullitions (1235): boiling or bubbling up

Ecchymoses (404): bruising

Empyreumatic (424): foul odor caused by decay

Epigastrium (925): upper central quadrant of the abdomen

Epistaxis (875): nosebleed

Eructations (98): belching.

Erysipelas (117): type of cellulitis, which is a superficial skin infection caused by Beta Hemolytic Strep

Erythema (887): redness

Exanthemata (612): skin eruption associated with fever

Excoriation (718): abrasions of the skin

Excrescence (547): eruption from the surface of the skin

Exostosis (289): bony overgrowth

Farinaceous (613): starchy food such as pasta or grains

Filamentous (537): thin and stringy

Fistula (240): abnormal passage between the surface of the skin and a body cavity

Formification (498): creepy crawling sensation like insects on the skin

Fulgurating Pains (1179): pains that are sudden and violent

Fungus Haematodes (1009): soft fungating, easily bleeding, and malignant cancer

Furfuraceous (831): dandruff like

Ganglia (1325): cysts attached to the sheath of a tendon

Gangrenous (405): death of tissue

Glairy (538): consistency of an egg white

Glans (678): head of the penis

Haemorrhage (825): bleeding

Hectic (1287): constant

Herpes Circinatus (369): form of herpes associated with severe itching and more severe herpetic outbreaks occurring mostly in children

Herpes Zoster (842): chicken pox or shingles

Hydrocephalus (356): accumulation of fluid in the ventricles of the brain, causing compression of the brain

Hydrothorax (1201): collection of water in the lungs

Hyperaesthesia (241): increased sensitivity to stimuli

Hypertrophy (241): excessive growth or enlargement

Hypochondrium (870): upper left and right quadrants of the abdomen

Hypogastrium (678): lower central quadrant of the abdomen

Ichorous Discharge (286): thin, pus-filled, and acrid

Ilium (664): groin or flank or the upper portion of the hip bone

Impetigo (888): a contagious skin infection that begins with vesicles and then crusts over

Incipient (879): beginning

Indolent (714): no tendency to heal

Induration (406): hardening of tissue

Influenza (1045): flu

Intermitting (866): coming and going

Lactation (1314): production of breast milk

Lardaceous (714): resembling lard (solid fat)

Leprous Spots Annular (999): round leprous eruptions

Leucorrhea (951): vaginal discharge

Lividity (978): paleness

Lupus (130): tuberculosis of the skin, causing red brown tubercles in patches around the nose and ears

Lymphatics (1018): lymph node

Maculae (888): small, round, discolored, and non elevated portion of the skin

Mammae (938): breasts

Mania a Potu (1253): another name for delirium tremens, or d.t.'s, a state of alcohol withdrawal

Meatus (285): opening

Melanosis (246): excess pigmentation

Metastasis (499): movement of symptoms from one location to another

Miliary (369): size and shape of millet seeds

Nates (617): buttocks

Necrosis (751): localized death of tissue

Neuralgic (1045): nerve like pain

Nodosity (379): knotlike swelling protruding from the bone

Noxious Effluvia (612): bad odor coming from decaying tissue

Occiput (356): back of the head

Oedema (132): swelling

Onanism (876) : premature withdrawal during intercourse (coitus interruptus)

Ophthalmia (1182): inflammation of the eye

Orgasm of Blood (841): rush of blood to the affected part

Papular (998): small circumscribed elevations of the skin

Paroxysmal (102): sudden

Parturition (282): childbirth

Patella (909): kneecap

Pectoral Muscles (472): muscles of the chest

Pedunculated (1340): on a stalk

Pemphigus (988): severe skin disease with blister formation that develops in crops

Perineum (718): area lying between the vagina and the rectum

Periostitis (446): inflammation of the lining of the bones of the teeth

Petechiae (878): small pinpoint spots of bleeding in the skin

Phagadenic (428): rapidly spreading destructive ulcer

Phlegmonous (373): suppurative (pus forming) inflammation of the subcutaneous connective tissue

Phthisis (1198): tuberculosis

Pituitious (879): associated with a mucous discharge

Polypus (316): benign polyps or growths

Prosopalgia (968): tic douloureux, a neuralgia of the face

Proud Flesh Surrounded by (446): fungus-like growths such as warts from the base

Psoriasis Diffusa (993): type of psoriasis that is severe and confluent

Pudendum (570): external genitalia

Puerperal (612): during childbirth

Purpura (415): bleeding under the skin, larger than petechiae

Purulent Discharge (332): pus-like quality to the discharge, indicating infection

Rhagades Eruptions (698): eruptions associated with cracks or fissures of the skin

Rheumatic (1045): worse cold and damp

Roseola (831): rose-colored eruption

Rupia (991): ulcers of late syphilis covered with yellow brown crusts similar in shape to oyster shells

Sacrum (564): tailbone

Scapula (515): shoulder blade

Schirrous Ulcer (82): ulcer that is cancerous and associated with much hard fibrous tissue

Scrobiculis Cordis (1264): pit of the stomach

Scorbutic (1319): related to vitamin C deficiency or scurvy

Scurfy (994): dandruff-like

Sequelae (747): aftermath

Serpiginous (714): healing on one side of a skin lesion while simultaneously extending on the other side

Smuttiness (1190): blackened or smudged

Sopor (768): stupor

Sordes (447): black crusts found during typhoid fever

Steatoma (319): fatty benign tumor

Sternum (902): breast bone

Stricture (467): narrowing or constriction

Submaxillary Glands (857): glands found under the tongue

Suppuration (117): pus-causing infection

Tetanic (968): steady muscular contractions

Tetter (983): another name for eczema

Thrombosis (1207): blood clot

Titillating (1317): tickling

Tonic (968): steady contraction of the muscles

Typhoid Fever (950): infectious disease causing high fevers, delirium, intestinal bleeding, skin eruption and diarrhea

Umbilicus (857): belly button

Undulating (844): wavy

Uremic (1235): accumulation of urinary products as a consequence of renal failure

Urticaria (768): hives

Varicella Like (987): blisters, like in chicken pox

Variola (809): chicken pox

Vertex (9378): top of the head

Vesicle (1322): small fluid-filled blisters

Vicarious (338): taking place instead of something else, such as menses

Wen (319): sebaceous cyst

APPENDIX I

Repetorization Case Template

CASE: **RUBRIC:**   **TOTAL**

Remedy	1	2	3	4	5	6	7	8	9	10
ABIES-C										
ACON										
ACT-S										
AESC										
AGAR										
ALL-C										
ALOE										
ALUMN										
AMBR										
AM-C										
AM-M										
ANAC										
ANT-C										
ANT-T										
APIS										
ARG-M										
ARG-N										
ARN										
ARS										
ARS-I										
ARUM-T										
AUR										
AUR-M										
BACC										
BAPT										
BAR-C										
BAR-M										
BELL										
BELLIS										
BEN-AC										
BERB										
BISM										
BOV										
BROM										
BRY										
CACT										
CALAD										
CALC-C										
CALC-F										
CALC-P										
CALC-S										
CAMPH										
CANN-I										
CANTH										
CAPS										
CARBO-A										
CARBO-V										
CAUL										
CAUST										
CHAM										
CHEL										
CHINA										

Remedy	1	2	3	4	5	6	7	8	9	10
CHIN-A										
CHIN-S										
CIMIC										
CINA										
CLEM										
COCC										
COFF										
COLCH										
COLOC										
CON										
CROT-H										
CROT-T										
CUPR										
CUPR-AR										
DIG										
DIOS										
DROS										
DULC										
EUP-PER										
EUPHR										
FERR										
FERR-AR										
FERR-P										
FL-AC										
GELAPS										
GLON										
GRAPH										
HAM										
HELL										
HEP										
HYDR										
HYOS										
HYPER										
IGN										
IOD										
IP										
IRIS										
KALI-AR										
KALI-BR										
KALI-C										
KALI-M										
KALI-P										
KALI-S										
KALM										
KREOS										
LAC-C										
LACH										
LAC-AC										
LED										
LIL-T										
LOB										
LYC										
MAG-C										
MAG-M										
MAG-P										
MAG-S										
MANG										
MED										

Remedy	1	2	3	4	5	6	7	8	9	10
MERC										
MERC-C										
MERC-IR										
MERC-IF										
MEZ										
MILL										
MUR-AC										
NAJA										
NAT-C										
NAT-M										
NAT-P										
NAT-S										
NIT-AC										
NUX-M										
NUX-V										
OP										
OX-AC										
PETRO										
PH-AC										
PHOS										
PHYT										
PIC-AC										
PIB										
PODO										
PSORN										
PULS										
PYROG										
RAN-B										
RHODO										
RHUS-T										
RUMEX										
RUTA										
SABAD										
SABIN										
SANG										
SEC										
SEL										
SEP										
SIL										
SPIG										
SPONG										
STANN										
STAPH										
STRAM										
STRONT										
STROPH										
SULPH										
SUL-AC										
SYPH										
TAB										
TARENT										
TEUCR										
THUJA										
TUB										
URT-U										
VERAT-A										
VERAT-V										
ZINC										

140

Source: National Center for Homeopathy

Sample Repetorization Case

CASE: John

Left table

RUBRIC	p.459	p.458	p.459	p.473	p.485	p.46				TOTAL
	1	2	3	4	5	6	7	8	9	10
ABIES-C										
ACON										
ACT-S										
AESC										
AGAR										
ALL-C										
ALOE				1						1
ALUMN										
AMBR										
AM-C										
AM-M										
ANAC										
ANT-C										
ANT-T										
APIS			2		1					3
ARG-M										
ARG-N										
ARN										
ARS				1						1
ARS-I										
ARUM-T										
AUR										
AUR-M										
BACC										
BAPT										
BAR-C										
BAR-M										
BELL	3				2					5
BELLIS										
BEN-AC										
BERB										
BISM										
BOV										
BROM		1								1
BRY				1						1
CACT										
CALAD										
CALC-C										
CALC-F										
CALC-P			1							1
CALC-S										
CAMPH										
CANN-I										
CANTH	1		1							2
CAPS										
CARBO-A										
CARBO-V										
CAUL										
CAUST										
CHAM										
CHEL			1							1
CHINA										

Middle table

RUBRIC	1	2	3	4	5	6	7	8	9	10
CHIN-A										
CHIN-S										
CIMIC						1				1
CINA										
CLEM										
COCC										
COFF										
COLCH										
COLOC										
CON										
CROT-H		2								2
CROT-T										
CUPR										
CUPR-AR										
DIG										
DIOS										
DROS										
DULC										
EUP-PER										
EUPHR										
FERR										
FERR-AR										
FERR-P										
FL-AC										
GELAPS				1						1
GLON						1				1
GRAPH										
HAM										
HELL										
HEP										
HYDR										
HYOS						2				2
HYPER										
IGN	1									1
IOD										
IP										
IRIS										
KALI-AR										
KALI-BR						1				1
KALI-C										
KALI-M										
KALI-P										
KALI-S										
KALM										
KREOS										
LAC-C										
LACH	3	3	3	1	1	2				13
LAC-AC										
LED										
LIL-T										
LOB										
LYC	2		2							4
MAG-C										
MAG-M										
MAG-P										
MAG-S										
MANG										
MED										

Right table

RUBRIC	1	2	3	4	5	6	7	8	9	10
MERC										
MERC-C	3									3
MERC-IR										
MERC-IF			1							1
MEZ										
MILL										
MUR-AC										
NAJA		1								1
NAT-C										
NAT-M						2				2
NAT-P										
NAT-S										
NIT-AC										
NUX-M										
NUX-V										
OP										
OX-AC										
PETRO										
PH-AC										
PHOS							1			1
PHYT			3							3
PIC-AC										
PIB							1			1
PODO										
PSORN										
PULS										
PYROG										
RAN-B										
RHODO										
RHUS-T							2			2
RUMEX										
RUTA										
SABAD						1				1
SABIN										
SANG										
SEC										
SEL										
SEP		1								1
SIL										
SPIG										
SPONG			1							1
STANN										
STAPH										
STRAM										
STRONT										
STROPH										
SULPH										
SUL-AC	1									1
SYPH										
TAB										
TARENT										
TEUCR		1								1
THUJA										
TUB										
URT-U										
VERAT-A										
VERAT-V							1			1
ZINC										

Layout of the Abdominal Section of the Repertory

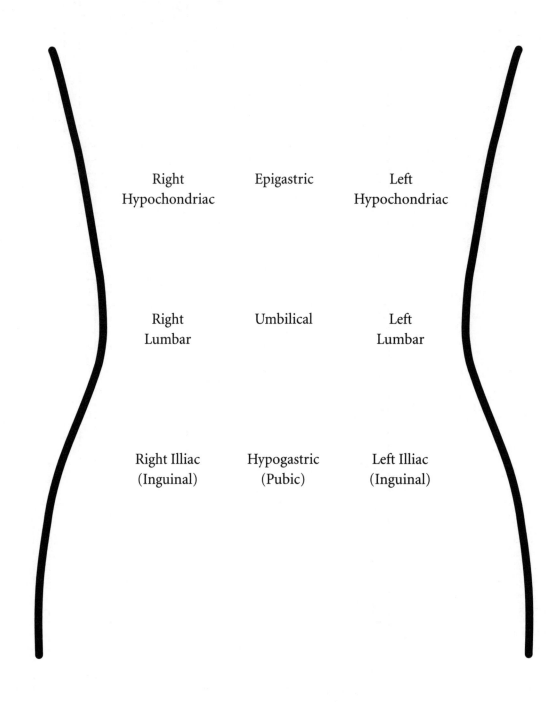

Right
Hypochondriac

Epigastric

Left
Hypochondriac

Right
Lumbar

Umbilical

Left
Lumbar

Right Illiac
(Inguinal)

Hypogastric
(Pubic)

Left Illiac
(Inguinal)

Answers to Quizzes

Answers to Quiz for Lesson One

1. D (Tendency to progress over time)
2. Nondirective questions; minimal initial questions followed by listening to the patient's story
3. Character, Location, Laterality, Time Aggravation, Weather, and Miscellaneous Factors
4. D (Fear of public speaking)
5. B (Headache during the full moon)
6. Position, Dreams, Drooling, Restlessness, Insomnia, Grinding Teeth, Talking in Sleep, Walking in Sleep, Desire to be Covered, Perspiration, Deep vs. Light Sleep, Unusual Movement, Desired Temperature, Emotional State on Waking, Refreshing vs. Unrefreshing

Answers to Quiz for Lesson Two

1. Temperature; Weather Sensitivity; Climate Preference; Energy; Sensitivity; Clothing; Bathing
2. B (Emotional level)
3. Center of Gravity, Age, Heredity, Sensitivity, and Suppression
4. Spontaneity, Clarity, Intensity, Frequency
5. No; the symptom of "Desires Pickles" is a side effect of the medication and is not indicative of the individual
6. Skin, Nervous, Digestive, Musculoskeletal, Urinary, Reproductive, Special Senses, Cardiovascular, Respiratory, Endocrine
7. An Obstacle to Cure is a factor in an individual's life that prevents them from moving forward to a greater level of health in treatment. This might include tobacco usage, abuse of alcohol, emotional abuse from a spouse, or dietary indiscretions.

Answers to Quiz for Lesson Four

1. *Nux vomica;* a single 30C potency was administered for three days and the symptoms completely resolved.

Nux vomica is one of our main remedies for colic in infants and children. There is often irritability and anger associated. Arching of the back is often noted with the colic. The stomach pains are worse from anger and better from warmth or warm drinks. The colic is often worse after eating and better from stool. Constipation is often present with hard, painful stools.

Below you will find a computer repetorization analysis of this case. In the numerical column called "Total," you will found a summation of all the numbers that lie below it. In the numerical column called "Rubrics," you will find the number of rubrics that appear for that particular remedy. The remedies that come up most strongly in the repetorization are found on the far left, followed by remedies in descending order of importance.

	Nux-v	Sulph.	Ars.	Phos.	Chin.	Sep.	Acon.	Bell.	Hep.	Kali-c.
TOTAL	14	10	7	6	5	5	4	4	4	4
RUBRICS	5	4	4	2	3	3	2	2	2	2
1. Sleep; WAKING; 3 a.m.	3	3	1		1	1				2
2. Mind; IMPATIENCE	3	3	2		1	3	2	1	2	2
3. Mind; SENSITIVE; light	3		2	3			2	3		
DESIRES; highly seasoned food	2	3		3	3	1			2	
Pain; General; warm; drinks amel.	3	1	2							

2. *Croton tiglium;* a single 30C potency was administered and the symptoms completed resolved within four hours

Croton tiglium is one of our main remedies for poison oak and poison ivy. The rash is vesicular and usually found on the face or genitals. Often the itching that is associated is described as intolerable. It is also an important gastrointestinal remedy and is commonly associated with diarrhea. Below you will find a computer repetorization analysis of the case.

	Crot-t.	Rhus-t.	Dulc.	Manc.	Calc-p.	Agar.	Merc.	Psor.	Sep.	Ant-c.
TOTAL	5	6	5	5	2	4	4	4	4	3
RUBRICS	3	2	2	2	2	2	2	2	2	2
1. Skin; ERUPTIONS; vesicular; yellow	1	3	3	2	1	2	2	1	1	1
2. Face; ERUPTIONS; vesicles	3	3	2	3		2	2	3	3	2
DIARRHOEA; alternating with; eruptions	1				1					

3. *Cocculus indica;* a single 30C potency was administered and the symptoms completely resolved in 24 hours

Cocculus indica is one of the major remedies for nausea and vomiting of pregnancy. It is also one of the most important remedies for motion sickness. Often there is vertigo associated. The nausea and vomiting is much worse with even the smell or thought of food. These patients can have great anxiety about others. It is said to be one of the main remedies for night watching. This is a condition where someone stays up late at night watching someone who is sick and thus becomes exhausted. There also may be thirst without a desire to drink. Below is a computer repertorization analysis of this case.

	Cocc.	Sep.	Ars.	Sulph.	Ip.	Phos.	Colch.	Nat-m	Kali-c	Lac-ac
TOTAL	8	8	6	6	6	4	5	5	5	5
RUBRICS	4	4	3	4	3	2	2	2	2	2
1. Stomach; NAUSEA; pregnancy during		3	2	1	2	2	2	2	2	3
2. Stomach; NAUSEA; motion, on	3	1		1	2				3	2
3. Stomach; NAUSEA; food; smell of	2	2	2		2		3			
4. Mind; ANXIETY; others for	1		2	2		2				
DWELLS on past disagreeable…	2	2		2				3		

4. C
5. B
6. D

Answers to Quiz for Lesson Five

1. Mind, Dipsomania (36)
2. Mind, Sensitive, Noise, Slightest (79)
*3. Mind, Timidity (88) (See note below)
4. Mind, Fastidious (42)
5. Mind, Suspiciousness (85)
6. Mind, Industrious, Mania for Work (56); Mind, Occupation, Amel (69); Mind, Busy (10); Mind, Work, Desire for Mental (95)
7. Mind, Conscientious about Trifles (16)
8. Mind, Flattery, Desires for (48)
9. Mind, Touched, Aversion to Being (89)
10. Mind, Fear, Happen, Something will (45)
11. Mind, Anger, Forenoon (2)
12. Mind, Eccentricity (39)
13. Mind, Sadness, Respiration, Impeded (77)

14. Mind, Recognize, Does not His Own House (71)
15. Mind, Suicidal Disposition, Shooting (85)
16. Mind, Delusions, God, Object of Divine Vengeance, He is the (26)
17. Mind, Anxiety of Conscience p. 6; Mind, Remorse (71)
18. Mind, Capriciousness p. 10; Mind Inconstancy (54)
19. Mind, Unconsciousness, after Emotion (90)
20. Mind, Loquacity (63)

*Note that what is important here is not the relationship (e.g., brother). What is important in finding the rubric is always the behavior.

Answers to Quiz for Lesson Six

1. Generalities, Side, Left (1401)
2. Generalities, Exertion Ameliorates (1358)
3. Generalities, Faintness, Pain from, in Teeth (1360)
4. Generalities, Pain, Appear Suddenly and Disappear Suddenly (1377)
5. Generalities, Narcotics Aggravate (1375)
6. Generalities, Menses, Before (1373)
7. Generalities, Pain, Soreness, Glands (1385)
8. Generalities, Chlorosis (1347)
9. Generalities, Ascending (1345)
10. Generalities, Heat, Flushes of (1365)
11. Generalities, Bathing Dread of (1345)
12. Generalities, Autumn (1345)
13. Generalities, Heat, Vital Lack of (1366)
14. Generalities, Air, Seashore, Ameliorates (1344)
15. Generalities, Night, Midnight, after, Ameliorates (1343)
16. Generalities, Tobacco Ameliorates (1407)
17. Generalities, Paralysis Agitans (1390)
18. Chest, Phthisis (878)
19. Generalities, Caged in Wire, Twisted Tighter and Tighter (1346)
20. Generalities, Convulsions, Excitement from (1353)

Answers to Quiz for Lesson Seven

1. Vision, Accommodation Defective (271); see also Vision, Loss of, Light By, Entering from Dark (282)
2. Ears, Discoloration, Redness, Evening (287)
3. Vertigo, Fall Tendency to, Right (99)
4. Face, Warts, Mouth Around (396)
5. Hearing, Impaired, Mortification after (323)
6. Mouth, Salivation, Sleep During (418)

7. Nose, Smell, Acute, Sensitive to the Odor of, Cooking Food (349)
8. Mouth, Fingers in the Mouth Children Put (405)
9. Head, Perspiration, Scalp, Sleep, During (222)
10. Head, Pain, after, Overeating, after (139)
11. Vision, Flickering, Morning, Waking (278)
12. Vision, Colors Before the Eyes, Green (274)
13. Head, Pain, Nail as From a, Vertex, three a.m. to four a.m. (188)
14. Vision, Loss of Vision, Headache, at Beginning of (282)
15. Eye, Inflammation, Conjunctiva (243)
16. Face, Cobwebs, Sensation of (356)
17. Mouth, Aphthae, Tongue, Tip (397)
18. Nose, Epistaxis, Vicarious (338)
19. Mouth, Taste, Metallic (424)
20. Head, Hair, Falling (120)

Answers to Quiz for Lesson Eight

1. Bladder, Urination, Involuntary, Night (659)
2. Stomach, Aversion, Eggs (480)
3. Larynx and Trachea, Voice, Lost (760)
4. Genitalia Female, Leucorrhea, Menses, after (722)
5. Genitalia, Condylomata, Scrotum (694)
6. Urine, Sediment, Renal Calculi (690)
7. Genitalia Female, Menses, Delayed in Girls First Menses (726)
8. Rectum, Constipation, Pregnancy During (608)
9. External Throat, Goiter, Right Sided (471)
10. Throat, Discoloration, Dark Red (450)
11. Thirst, Unquenchable (530)
12. Stomach, Nausea, Beer after (506)
13. Abdomen, Inflammation, Appendicitis (552)
14. Teeth, Pain, Autumn in the (435)
15. Bladder, Retention of Urine, Enlarged Prostate, from (651)
16. Abdomen, Rumbling (600)
17. Rectum, Haemorrhoids, Internal (620)
18. Stool, Lenteric (638)
19. Stomach, Desires, Indigestible Things Mouth (485)
20. Teeth, Dentition, Slow (431)

Answers to Quiz for Lesson Nine

1. Chest, Palpitation, Excitement after (875)
2. Back, Opisthonos (893)

3. Cough, Inspiration (794)
4. Sleep, Dreams, Events of the Previous Day, Long Past (1239)
5. Extremities, Awkwardness (953)
6. Back, Coldness, Cervical Region (886)
7. Extremities, Cold, Foot, Icy (963)
8. Sleep, Dreams, Nightmares (1242)
9. Perspiration, Profuse, Night (1299)
10. Extremities, Discoloration, Fingers, Nails, White, Spots (981)
11. Extremities, Restlessness, Leg, Sleep During (1188)
12. Skin, Stings of Insects (1331); see also p. 1368
13. Chest, Formification, Axilla in (832)
14. Skin, Discoloration, Red, Scratching, Streaks after (1306)
15. Chill, Tertian (1273)
16. Sleep, Position, Side On, Left, Impossible (1247)
17. Sleep, Yawning, Eating after (1257)
18. Skin, Eruptions, Herpetic, Zoster Zona (1314)
19. Cough, Sympathetic (807)
20. Extremities, Cramps, Calf, Night (975)

Answers to Quiz for Lesson Ten

1. D
2. C (Sycotic Miasm)
3. B (Plants)
4. C (Common symptom)
5. D (Sepia, Nux Vomica, Sulphur)
6. C (Characteristic symptoms)
7. D (Etiology)
8. E (Pathology)

Answers to Practice Cases

The repetorizations listed below are done using a computerized program called McRepertory. The number in the totals column is the sum of all the numbers in the column below. The number in the rubrics column is the number of rubrics that the particular remedy appears in.

1. Important symptoms here include the etiology (a puncture wound), swelling, bruising, and coldness ameliorates. The one strange, rare, and peculiar symptom here is "chilly and yet better when cold."

	Led.	Puls.	Arn.	Lach.	Phos.	Apis.	Carb-v.	Sulph.	Nit-ac.	Bry.	Sec.
TOTAL	14	10	8	8	8	8	7	7	7	7	7
RUBRICS	5	4	4	4	4	3	5	5	4	3	3
1. Generalities; WOUNDS	3	2	2	2	2	2	1	1	1		
WOUNDS; penetrating	3					3	2	1	3		
3. Extremities; SWELLING; Foot	3	3	2	2	2	3	1	1	2	3	2
4. Skin; ECCHYMOSES	3	2	3	2	3		2	2		2	3
COLD; becoming; amel.	2	3	1	2	1		1	2	1	2	2

He was given *Ledum palustre* 30C in a single dose. Within twelve hours all the symptoms resolved and there was no recurrence of any symptoms.

Ledum is the most important remedy for puncture wounds. *Hypericum perfoliatum* and *Apis mellifica* are other important remedies. *Ledum* is associated with much swelling and a blue-purple appearance to the wound. It also has the characteristic keynote of "chilly and yet better cold." *Ledum* can also help with cellulitis (superficial skin infections).

2. Important symptoms here are the suddenness of the onset of the pain and the severity of symptoms. The pain is burning and there is tenesmus. There also is much blood. Her moods reflect the violence of the onset and the irritability of her system.

	Canth.	Lyc.	Puls.	Apis.	Ter.	Ars.	Caps.	Nux-v.	Acon.	Bell.	Sep.
TOTAL	14	12	12	11	11	10	10	10	10	9	9
RUBRICS	6	6	5	5	4	5	5	5	4	4	4
1. Bladder; INFLAMMATION	3	3	3	3	3	2	2	2	3	3	3
2. Bladder; PAIN; burning	3	1	2	2	3	2	3	1	2	1	2
PAIN; burning; urination; during	2	1			2		1	1			
4. Bladder; TENESMUS	3	2	3	2	3	3	2	3	2	2	1
5. Urine; BLOODY; clots	1	2	1	1		1					
6. Mind; IRRITABILITY	2	3	3	3		2	2	3	3	3	3

She was given two doses of *Cantharis vesicatoria* 30C four hours apart. Symptoms gradually improved and within twelve hours there was complete resolution of all symptoms, with no recurrence.

Cantharis is one of the main remedies for urinary tract infections. Infections are characteristically sudden and violent. There is often a great deal of burning associated, as well as tenesmus (cramping). There is also much blood and clotting. Emotionally, there is often great irritability and intensity. Untreated, these infections often evolve into kidney infections (pyelonephritis).

3. This is a deeper case. The key symptoms in this case relate to the sleepiness and significant impairment in her breathing. The rattling respiration and winter aggravation are also strong.

	Ars.	Carb-v.	Phos.	Hep.	Puls.	Ant-t.	Caust.	Lyc.	Nux-v.	Sil.	Sulph.
TOTAL	16	14	14	13	13	13	12	12	12	12	11
RUBRICS	6	6	6	6	6	5	6	6	6	6	6
1. Generalities; WINTER, in	2	1	2	2	1		2	1	3	2	1
2. Generalities; CYANOSIS	2	3	1	1	1	2	1	1	1	1	1
3. Respiration; RATTLING	3	2	3	3	3	3	3	3	2	2	2
DIFFICULT; lying, while	3	3	2	2	2	2	1	2	1	2	2
5. Sleep; SLEEPINESS	3	3	3	2	3	3	3	2	3	2	3
INFLAMMATION; Bronchial tubes	3	2	3	3	3	3	2	3	2	3	2

She was given *Antimonium tartaricum* 30C daily for five days. Symptoms gradually improved over the course of the next week. The bronchitis resolved within seven days. Her breathing continued to improve and she was able to get off of oxygen completely and became much more functional than she ever had been over the winter. Following the treatment, she had no further recurrences of bronchitis.

The remedy given here was not the most prominent remedy in the repetorization. Remember that the repertory is only a tool and ultimately serves as a suggestion to what remedies to study . Ultimately the remedy choices rely far more on the materia medica.

Antimonium tartaricum is an important remedy for bronchitis, especially of the elderly. There is much rattling of the respiration. There is frequently a cough, which is not productive, although they struggle greatly to cough up mucus. There tends to be severe respiratory problems and a weakened depleted state. There is often blueness and cyanosis. Sleepiness is characteristic. Symptoms are typically worse when lying down and worse in a warm room.

4. This is a case of croup. What is characteristic about the case is the time aggravation modality, the aggravation from cold drinks, and the amelioration from hot drinks. The anxiety and swollen lymph nodes are quite typical of this condition and probably should not be used as symptoms.

	Spong.	Ars.	Phos.	Hep.	Acon.	Bell.	Brom.	Calc.	Carb-v.	Iod.	Lach.
TOTAL	14	13	13	12	10	10	10	10	10	10	10
RUBRICS	6	5	5	5	4	4	4	4	4	4	4
1. Generalities; WINTER, in	3	2	3	3	3	2	2			3	3
2. Generalities; CYANOSIS	3	3	3	2	3	3	3	3	2	3	3
3. Respiration; RATTLING	1	3	2	3	1	2	2	3	3	1	1
DIFFICULT; lying, while	2										
5. Sleep; SLEEPINESS	2	3	2	1				1	2		
INFLAMMATION; Bronchial tubes	3	2	3	3	3	3	3	3	3	3	3

She was given *Spongia tosta* 30C in two doses six hours apart. The symptoms resolved completely in twelve hours.

Spongia is one of the main remedies for croup. *Aconite napellus, Hepar sulphuris* and *Sulphur* are the other main remedies. The *Spongia* cough is typically dry, and worse before midnight. It is better with hot drinks and worse with cold drinks. It is described as tickling, and there is a feeling of dryness in the throat. Often there is hoarseness associated.

5. Key symptoms in this case are the severe bandlike headaches radiating over the top of the head. There is dullness and depression associated. There are problems with visual accommodation. The tremor is also unusual.

	Gels.	Nat-m.	Arg-n.	Sulph.	Calc.	Cocc.	Merc.	Sil.
TOTAL	17	16	11	11	11	10	10	10
RUBRICS	7	7	5	5	4	5	5	4
LOCALIZATION; Occiput; extending; forehead, to	3	2	2	1	2		1	2
2. Vertigo; HEADACHE, during	2	2	2	1	3	2	2	3
3. Generalities; MORNING; 10 a.m.	1	3						
4. Head; CONSTRICTION; band or hoop	3	1	2	3		2	2	
5.Mind; DULLNESS	3	3	3	3	3	2	2	3
6. Extremities; TREMBLING; Hand	2	3	2	3	3	2	3	2
7. Vision; ACCOMMODATION; slow	3	2				2		

She was given *Gelsemium sempervirens* 30C daily for three days. Her symptoms completely resolved over that time and there was no recurrence.

Gelsemium is one of the best remedies for headaches. They tend to be severe and spread from the occiput to the forehead, and are often associated with a band sensation. There is also much dizziness associated with this remedy. There is a ten a.m., time aggravation. There is much weakness and depletion associated with the remedy, including trembling. Patients are often described as dull, depressed and dizzy.

6. The most important thing in this case is the etiology, "worse cold and damp." What is characteristic is the "better with warm drinks" and the improvement in symptoms after talking. There is severe lower back pain and restlessness associated. The sore throat is to be expected and should not be used as a symptom.

	Rhus-t.	Ars.	Lyc.	Nux-v.	Chin.	Dulc.
TOTAL	15	13	11	11	11	10
RUBRICS	6	5	5	5	4	4
1. Throat; PAIN; Sorethroat; warm; drinks; amel.	2	3	3	1		
VOICE; hoarseness; talking; a while, improves after	2					
3. Generalities; HEAT; vital, lack of	3	3	2	3	2	3
4. Back; PAIN; Backache; Lumbar region	3	1	1	3	3	3
5. Extremities; RESTLESSNESS	3	3	3	3	3	2
6. Stomach; DESIRES; cold drinks	2	3	2	1	3	2

He was given *Rhus toxicodendron* 30C in a single dose. Symptoms resolved completely within three hours. There was no recurrence of symptoms.

Rhus toxicodendron is a remedy often forgotten for influenza. One of the main characteristics is "worse when cold and damp." It also has the characteristic of being better from motion. Once the throat warms up, it improves. There is often restlessness associated with the complaints.

7. This is a case of dysmenorrhea. Characteristic symptoms include the simultaneous vomiting and diarrhea and the great chilliness and perspiration. The coldness also extends to Raynaud's Syndrome. There is a strong craving for salt. The actual dysmenorrhea symptoms are not particularly characteristic.

	Verat.	Arg-n.	Calc.	Carb-v	Nux-v.	Puls.
TOTAL	14	11	11	11	11	10
RUBRICS	5	5	4	4	4	4
1. Female Genitalia; PAIN; Uterus; menses; during			3		3	3
2. Stomach; VOMITING; General; diarrhoea; during	3	3				2
3. Perspiration; PROFUSE	3	1	3	3	2	2
4. Generalities; MORNING	2	2	3	3	3	3
EXtremities; COLDNESS; Hands; icy	3	2		2	2	
6. Stomach; DESIRES; salty things	3	3	2	3		

She took *Veratrum album* 12C daily for six weeks. Her first period after the remedy was started showed moderate improvement and the next period showed complete resolution of symptoms. There was no recurrence. The chilliness also resolved completely with treatment.

Veratrum album is an important remedy for dysmenorrhea, especially in adolescents. A characteristic keynote is the simultaneous vomiting and diarrhea. There is great chilliness and perspiration. It is one of the main remedies for Raynaud's Syndrome. There is often a strong craving for salt, ice, and fruit.

8. This is another case of influenza. What is characteristic here is the confusion and sleepiness. There is also a high fever. The foul odor is very strong. She has busy dreams.

	Bapt.	Bry.	Lach.	Sil.	Carb-v.	Rhus-t
TOTAL	14	11	11	11	11	10
RUBRICS	7	6	6	5	4	6
1. Mind; DULLNESS	3	3	3	3	3	2
2. Mind; CONFUSION	2	3	3	3	3	3
3. Mouth; ODOR; offensive	2	2	3	1	3	1
4. Sleep; DREAMS; busy	1	3	1			
5. Generalities; HARD bed, sensation of	2	1		3		2
6. Stool; ODOR; putrid	3	2	2	3	3	1
7. Throat; DISCOLORATION; redness; dark red	3		2			2

She was given a single dosage of *Baptisia tinctoria* 200C. Symptoms resolved completely within twelve hours. There was no further recurrence of symptoms.

Baptisia is a remedy that is associated with great confusion and dullness of the mind. There tend to be high fevers. It is an important remedy for influenza. Associated with the symptoms are putrid odors. The throat itself shows a dark red inflammation, which is pain-free. Patients may have difficulty swallowing, especially solids. Another keynote for this remedy is feeling bruised all over and the bed feeling too hard. The dreams are quite busy.

9. There is little that is individuating here about the actual infection. What is more characteristic are the mental symptoms. He cannot be satisfied and does not want to be touched. His whole nervous system is wound up. Another strange symptom is the crying in sleep at night.

	Cham.	Puls.	Bell.	Sulph.	Lyc.	Kali-c.	Merc.	Calc.	Bry.	Nat-m.	Dulc.
TOTAL	22	17	15	15	13	12	12	11	11	11	10
RUBRICS	8	7	7	6	6	5	5	7	6	5	6
1. Ear; INFLAMMATION; media	3	3	2	3	3	2	3	3		2	2
2. Mind; SHRIEKING; pain, with the	3	1	3								
3. Mind; CAPRICIOUSNESS	3	2	2	2	1	3		1	3		2
4. Mind; DISCONTENTED	2	2	1	3	2	2	3	1	2	3	1
5. Mind; TOUCHED; aversion to being	3		2			3	1	1	2		
6. Mind; SHRIEKING; sleep, during	2	3		2	3			1	2	1	1
7. Stool; GREEN	3	3	2	3	2		3	2	1	3	2
8. Ear; PAIN; General; inside	3	3	3	2	2	2	2	2	1	2	2

He was given a single dosage of *Chamomilla* 30C. No further dosages were needed. There was no further recurrence of symptoms.

Chamomilla is a remedy that has great hypersensitivity and a wound-up nervous system. It is one of our best remedies for ear infections. There tends to be great dissatisfaction, capriciousness, and shrieking. This even comes out in the sleep. There is great sensitivity to pain. There is a focus also on the gastrointestinal tract, with colic and green stools.

10. This is a case of bronchitis. What is characteristic about this case is the severe, intractable vomiting.

	Ip.	Phos.	Arg-n.	Ars.	Acon.	Bry.	kali-c.	Puls.	Dig.
TOTAL	12	12	11	11	10	10	10	10	8
RUBRICS	5	5	5	4	5	4	4	4	5
INFLAMMATION; Bronchial tubes; children	3						3		
2. Respiration; ASTHMATIC	3	2	3	3	2	2	3	3	2
3. Stomach; VOMITING; General; incessant	2	2	2	2					1
4. Expectoration; BLOODY, spitting of blood	3	3	2	3	3	2	1	3	2
5. Generalities; HEATED, becoming	1	2	2		1	3	3	3	2
6. Stomach; DESIRES; cold drinks		3	2	3	3	3		1	1

She was treated with *Ipecacuanha* 30C for three doses every four hours over a twelve hour period. The symptoms gradually resolved over that period. There was no recurrence of symptoms afterwards.

Ipecacuanha is an important remedy for bronchitis, particularly in children. It can also be a remedy for croup and whooping cough. There tends to be severe nausea and vomiting associated. There also is a strong bleeding tendency. It tends to be a warm remedy. It is also a major remedy for migraine headaches.

Glossary of Homeopathic Terms

Acute: self-limited, characterized by a latent period, a period of exacerbation, and then a period of decline of symptoms, which may result in cure or death

Aggravation: an increase of symptoms experienced by the patient after taking the remedy, followed by a truly curative response

Allopathy: system of medicine wherein prescribed medicines have symptoms that have no direct relationship to the disease condition; symptoms neither similar nor opposite but completely heterogenous

Antidote: any substance, energetic stimulus, or procedure that clearly stops the curative action of a homeopathic remedy

Center of Gravity: a measure of the patient's illness based on the intensity of the symptoms and the level of the hierarchical disturbance

Complementary: the relationship between two homeopathic remedies wherein the second of the two remedies follows the action of the first remedy, bringing the patient to cure

Concomitant: two symptoms occurring at the same time but without any pathological basis to their relationship or appearance; an example would be tooth pain and simultaneous elbow pain

Confirmatory: a symptom that confirms or validates the choice of a particular homeopathic remedy under consideration for prescription during the interview

Constitutional: a remedy that treats the whole person on all levels of their being

Cure: the disappearance of symptoms followed by a significant restoration of health and elimination of all the perceptible signs and symptoms of the disease; means also the removal of the inner modification of the vital force that underlies it

Delusion: a false perception of reality

Disease: deviation from the healthy condition as expressed through symptoms

Disruption: a substance that temporarily interferes with the curative action of a homeopathic remedy

Emotionals: a type of homeopathic symptom on one of the planes of homeopathic health (also physicals, mentals, generals)

Enantiopathy: a system of medicine wherein medications/treatments are based on prescribing for the direct opposite of the symptom

Engrafting: a process that allows proving symptoms to become a fixed part of a person's symptoms

Essence: that which is most characteristic, important, and essential about a remedy

Generals: symptoms that reflect the whole person rather than a single part

Health: freedom from pain in the physical body, having attained a state of well-being; freedom from excessive passion on the emotional level, having as a result reached a dynamic state of serenity and calm and freedom from selfishness in the mental sphere, having, as a result, connection with Truth; the measurement of health is creativity to promote continuous and unconditional happiness; it signifies freedom, spontaneity, and being in the present

Hering's Laws of Cure: Healing takes place from the interior to the exterior, from the center to the circumference, from above downward, from within outwards, from the most important to the less important organs

Homeopathy: a system of medicine founded by Dr. Samuel Hahnemann, based on:

1. The law of similars wherein a medicine that produces symptoms in a healthy human being is capable of curing any illness that displays similar effects

2. Potentization and minimum dose; homeopathic medicines are prepared by a process of dilution and succussion which creates an infinitesimal dose in a dynamized "potentized" form

Imponderabilia: remedies without substance (e.g., X-ray, Magnet, Electricity, Moon, Sun)

Inimical: homeopathic remedies that are theoretically antagonistic and will antidote the action of the first remedy

Isopathy: treating a disease with the identical substance that produced it (e.g., allergy shots)

Keynote: specific symptoms of a homeopathic remedy making it very unique and identifiable from other homeopathic remedies

Materia Medica: book(s) containing the compilation of reported symptoms from homeopathic drug proving and cured symptoms reported from clinical practice arranged by organ system

Medicine: a substance that can cure disease only by possessing the power to alter the way a person feels and functions

Mental State: refers to the disposition of the patient

Mental Symptom: refers to a symptom that can be described in the repertory but does not necessarily contain the "mental state" of the patient

Miasm: concept developed by Hahnemann to account for chronic disease states, in which the constitution of the person was weakened and the internal economy became disordered; Hahnemann concluded that this weakness could be transmitted from generation to generation; Kent discussed the problem as the first sickness of the human race (a spiritual sickness)

Modality: a modifier used in conjunction with a symptom (e.g., headache worse when cold)

Nosode: homeopathic remedy made from a disease product (e.g., *Tuberculinum* is made from tubercular tissue)

Obstacles to Cure: substances or situations that will block the action of a well prescribed remedy and prevent the patient from achieving restoration of health or cure

Pathology: a limitation of freedom on any of the planes of being

Planes: physical, emotional, mental, spiritual; readily identifiable hierarchy of construction in the human being, not separate and distinct but with a complete interaction between them

Polychrest: a remedy that is well proven, symptoms having being recorded in all systems of the body; a remedy often prescribed in clinical practice

Potency: refers to the strength of a homeopathic remedy

> **C:** homeopathic remedies prepared by diluting the substance in a serial dilution of 1 to 100 (centesimal=C=100) followed by succussion

> **X:** homeopathic remedies prepared by diluting the substance in a serial dilution of 1 to 10 (decimal=x=10=D) followed by succussion

> **M:** 1,000C

> **LM:** the last potency scale developed by Hahnemann; homeopathic remedies prepared by an initial 1 to 50,000 dilution followed by succussion; Hahnemann believed that this potency would permit more gentle treatment with less aggravations

Proving: homeopathic drug testing on healthy volunteers where symptoms that develop are recorded, compiled, and organized into a materia medica and repertory

Remedy: the individual homeopathic medicine

Repertory: a book of symptoms associated with listings of remedies categorized into different systems of the body

Restoration of Health: the re-establishment of order within the patient

Rubric: an individual entry in a repertory that describes a symptom

Sarcodes: homeopathic remedies made from healthy tissues or secretions

Similimum: the exactly right homeopathic remedy

SRP: strange, rare and peculiar; symptoms so unique and unusual that then bring to mind only a very limited number of remedies to be considered in the case

Succussion: a series of vigorous shakes

Suppression: any medicinal treatment causing symptoms to disappear but without restoring health or cure to the patient

Symptom: any expression of the basic function of the human being that occupies the attention of the person; any sensation that reminds the person of his bodily parts

Totality of Symptoms: the symptoms in each particular case of disease as expressed by the symptom's perceptible signs representing the entire extent of the sickness; the outer image expressing the inner essence of the disease of the disturbed vital force

Trituration: process where substances that are insoluble in alcohol are brought to the 3C potency by grinding the substance with milk sugar in a mortar and pestle for a total of three hours

Vital Force: the spiritlike dynamism that flows through the material human organism

"<": homeopathic shorthand indicating that whatever symptoms follow are worse from

">": homeopathic shorthand indicating that whatever symptoms follow are better from